Gout

The Ultimate Guide

Everything You Must Know About Gout

©All Rights Reserved

HR Research Alliance

This study aid is not intended to be any type of Medical advice. ALL individuals must consult their Doctors first and should always receive their meal plans from a qualified practitioner. This book is not intended to heal, or cure anyone from any kind of illness, or disease.

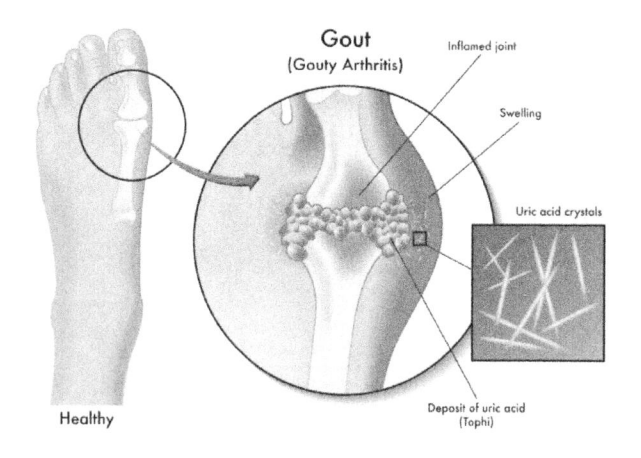

Table of Contents

Introduction 10

History of Gout 11

Gout Risk Factors 13

What Is Gout? 17

Stages of Gout 22

Causes of Gout 26

Gout Causing Foods 28

Lifestyle factors 31

Lifestyle triggers of gout 32

Symptoms of Gout 33

Diagnosing Gout 38

Alternative Therapies for Gout 51

Gout Diet 57

Foods to Avoid: 59

Lifestyle Changes for Gout 66

Prevention Strategy 76

Summary of Latest Gout Research 81

Apple Pie: Apple, Cinnamon, Almond 93

Beet the Rush Smoothie: Beet, Strawberry, Raspberry 94

Watermelon-Basil Lemonade: Watermelon, Strawberry, Basil 96

Creamy Cantaloupe: Cantaloupe, Pineapple, Banana 97

Peary-Cherry: Pear, Cherry 98

Peaches and Green: Peach & Avocado 99

Sweet Potato Pie: Sweet potato & Banana 100

Sweet Peach Tea: Peach, Green Tea 101

Sparkling Peach Spritzer: Peach, Grape 102

Cherry Citrus Smoothie: Pineapple, Cherry 103

Sunrise Smoothie: Kiwi, Watermelon, Strawberry 104

Better Birthday Cake: Vanilla, Spinach, Banana 105

Blue Raspberry Tea: Blueberry, Raspberry, White Tea 106

Blackberry Mango Tango: Blackberry, Mango, Honeydew 108

Mango Berry Smoothie: Mango, Blueberry 109

You've Broc-To Be Kidding: Broccoli, Blueberry, Orange 110

Blackberry Cobbler: Blackberry, Almond 111

Tasty and Refreshing Pineapple Avocado Smoothie 112

Tropical Pineapple Orange Smoothie 113

Delicious Kale Banana Smoothie 114

115

Easy Watermelon Strawberry Smoothie 116

Energetic Lime Watermelon Smoothie 117

Zinger Papaya Ginger Smoothie 118

Fresh Tropical Smoothie 119

Yummy Chocó Banana Smoothie 120

Cool and Creamy Pumpkin Banana Smoothie 121

Simple Mix Berry Smoothie 122

Healthy Immune Booster Smoothie 123

Pink Grapefruit Raspberry Smoothie 124

Green Grape Avocado Smoothie 125

Blueberry Chia Cherry Smoothie 126

Refreshing Apple Beet Smoothie 127

Choco Cherry Smoothie 128

Refreshing Melon Mint Smoothie 129

Hello, my name is Steven, and I have been dealing with gout, for close to 2 decades now. I have managed to keep it under control, by a few simple lifestyle, and diet changes, that have made my life overall a better one.

There are so many types, and severities of arthritis pains, and each individual will have different experiences with them.

While my gout has always been somewhat minor in comparison to others in my immediate family. I have had times, especially in the beginning, where it was painful to walk.

I want to encourage each individual who may be dealing with gout, to always consult with your practitioner. And understand that each person will have to change certain things in their lifestyle, depending on the severity of their pains.

While I am no expert on gout, nor do I make any claims to be. What I am an expert on (now), is the understanding of my own body. And what I can, and cannot eat, in order to not have flair ups.

I encourage you to also become an expert on your own body as well. Work with your Doctor, to find the right lifestyle that fits you perfectly. In order to live a healthy, pain free life.

I would like to share with you, some of my own thoughts, based on my years of researching the subject. And testing out certain types of eating patterns for my own self.

Gout does not have to keep us from enjoying our food, or our lives.

I wish you all the best, and know that you will too one day be an expert on what your body needs to feel its best.

I hope my experiences can help you out just a little. And I hope your experiences can do the same for someone as well.

Thank you
Steven

Introduction

You wake up one morning and notice your big toe is swollen, red, and sore. "What's going on," you think to yourself? You can't even think about walking right now, much less putting a shoe on your foot!

The pain of a gout attack is almost indescribable. It can come on suddenly overnight and you may even be terrified because the pain is so bad.

Gout is a form of arthritis that comes out of nowhere. The pain usually starts around 12 hours after the attack begins. In most cases, it hits the big toe first.

It may not even be your big toe. It tends to start in one joint, with the big toe being the joint in about half of the cases. Some experience the initial pain in a hand, ankle, or even the knee. All you know is the pain is one of the worst you have ever felt!

These symptoms may be new to you, but actually gout is thought to be a very ancient condition. Let's take a quick look at the history of gout.

History of Gout

Gout actually has quite the history and often called "the disease of kings." Dating as far back as the 5th century B.C., there are some accounts that aristocrats may have suffered from this condition due to diet. Gout is more common in those who eat heavy foods and drink alcohol. Some of the notable people who suffered from gout historically were:

King Henry VIII of England

Michelangelo

Christopher Columbus

Alexander the Great

Leonardo da Vinci

Sir Isaac Newton

Charles Dickens

Beethoven

Ben Franklin

While in the early days, it was known as the "unwalkable disease" and attributed to an imbalance, they had no idea what the imbalance was. Now, we know that it is high uric acid levels we're able to link this to excesses of certain foods in the diet, known as "high purine foods." These foods in ancient times were usually only eaten by wealthy kings.

Nowadays, we are able to afford most foods and the evidence of gout is on the rise in most of the general population. Wealthy or not.

Gout Statistics

Gout affects around 3.9% of the population in the U.S. This is over 8 million people. The growth of this condition is astounding to say the least. Back in the 1990's, gout affected around 2.7% of the population. Even those who aren't diagnosed with gout sometimes have signs they may develop gout in the future. Studies show that 21% of people in the United States have elevated uric acid levels, which is one of the main factors in gout.

Gout Risk Factors

As with any type of arthritis, there are increased risk factors for gout. Researchers have looked at gout from just about every angle and have found that it's not only related to what you eat and drink, but a whole range of factors:

High Purine Diet

Alcohol Intake (Especially Beer)

Organ Meat Intake

Increased Seafood Intake

High Fructose Foods

Certain Diuretics

History of Hypertension

Obesity

High Cholesterol

Diabetes

Genetics and Family History of Gout

A word about obesity. Out of all the risk factors listed above, being overweight can affect gout in a few different ways.

First, it increases the risk of getting gout. If you have a group of conditions known as, metabolic syndrome, you may be at a higher risk of gout. People who are obese and suffer from; high blood sugar, insulin sensitivity, obesity, and high blood pressure all tend to have higher uric acid levels.

Second, it can severely affect the pain of gout. Excessive weight puts pressure on irritated joints and can make it even harder to perform your daily tasks.

Third, being overweight increases complications. Being overweight can increase your risk of complications from gout. Increased stress on damaged joints, high cholesterol, high blood sugar, and high uric acid levels can be a deadly mix.

Age Range, Gender, and Ethnicity

Gout affects people in a certain age range, tends to affect more males than women, and is common in certain races of people. The numbers are as follows:

Age. As if the aches and pains of middle age aren't enough, throw in the possibility of gout in people who are ages 40 to 70. While most gout cases occur in males, out of those cases:

3.5% are women in the 60 to 69-year age bracket

4.6% occur in women aged 70 to 79

5.6% are women who are over 80 years of age

86.3% are men aged 65 to 84

Gender. Gout does tend to affect males more often than females. However, after a woman has reached menopause and the estrogen levels drop, the incidence of gout rises in women. Researchers have found that estrogen may help to regulate uric acid levels.

Ethnicity. While gout can affect anyone of any race, there does tend to be a higher number of gout sufferers in; African American, Asians, and Pacific Islanders. A surprising number is the Maori population in New Zealand, where 10% of the male population over the age of 20 suffer from gout.

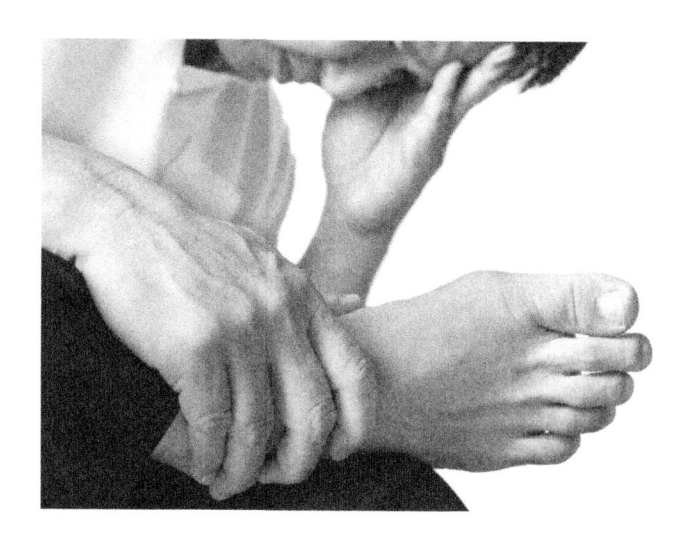

What Is Gout?

In a nutshell, gout is a type of arthritis. It is similar to, but different from rheumatoid arthritis, but we'll take a look at that later.

Gout or sometimes called "gouty arthritis," occurs when your body produces unusually high amounts of uric acid. Your kidneys may not excrete excess uric acid well and the levels rise in your blood. It is a severely painful type of arthritis, because excess uric acid forms into crystals. These crystals have a structure like needles and they "stab" into the joints and soft tissues of your body. Uric acid crystals irritate your tissues leading to inflammation and swelling.

Uric acid comes from purines in the diet. Purines are highest in; organ meats, canned mackerel, anchovies, sardines, dried legumes, and beer. If you are eating these things in moderation and have no risk factors for gout, your body breaks down the uric acid and leaves your body via your kidneys. If this process doesn't happen you develop elevated uric acid levels known as, hyperuricemia.

A large number of people who suffer from gout feel it in their great toe. In a smaller number of people, gout may affect other joints in the body such as; your knees, wrists, elbows, ankles and fingers.

Over time, the uric acid crystals can build up near the joints and you will notice lumps under your skin. These are called, tophi. If you squeeze the soft cartilage on your ears you may feel them. These crystals can also cause kidney stones. You can also develop "tophi" in your eyes, earlobes, soft tissues of the fingers, and even your lungs.

One of the differences between rheumatoid arthritis and gout is that gout occurs in episodes. You may have a "gout flare" that lasts up to a few weeks, and the symptoms can subside for a while and come back. Rheumatoid arthritis is a chronic condition where some level of symptoms tend to be present at all times. There are a few ways to tell the difference.

How do I know it's not rheumatoid arthritis?

After the initial attack, recurrent attacks can actually begin to look and feel like rheumatoid arthritis. So much that you may actually question which type you really have. In a few cases, people with gout may even test positive for the rheumatoid factor. This is an antibody your body produces when you are having a rheumatoid flare. Rheumatoid arthritis can also cause nodules under your skin that are similar to tophi. Even some doctors have questioned a diagnosis based on these two things. But what is it really?

When it comes to rheumatoid arthritis and gout, the two are actually quite different:

Sign	Gout	Rheumatoid Arthritis
Joint Pain and Swelling	x	x
Sudden Onset	x	
Positive Rheumatoid Factor	Possible	x
Flares/Episodes	x	
Chronic Joint Pain	Later in the Disease	x

Each has its own unique cause, explained here:

Rheumatoid Arthritis – In RA, your body produces antibodies that attack your joints. Your immune system sees something in your joints as foreign and sends out these antibodies to attack thinking there is an infection when there really is none. These attacks damage the joints and are chronic from the beginning.

Gout – Gout occurs from the buildup of uric acid crystals in the joints. When you have your first attack, the uric acid levels have been rising in your body and you may not have known it. The first attack comes on suddenly and eventually subsides and you will feel better for months to years before the next attack.

We will cover testing for gout in a bit, but there are some simple tests your doctor can do to differentiate between the two and make sure you get the proper treatment.

Stages of Gout

Gout happens in stages. It is considered a progressive condition, but very manageable with medications. It begins with the first stage, where you won't even know you have gout and progresses through the fourth stage or chronic gout.

Here is how each stage looks:

First Stage: Asymptomatic Gout

In the first stage of gout, you won't even know it's there. The uric acid levels begin to rise in your body, but don't cause any symptoms yet. It is possible to have high levels of uric acid and never progress to the second stage. Just know that it can take years between developing high uric acid levels and experiencing your first attack. Whether you are at risk or not for gout, if you have high uric acid levels you need to take steps to reduce it. You can ask your doctor for a simple test if you are at risk at your yearly check-up.

Second Stage: Acute Attack

This is the sudden and intense onset of pain and swelling. The uric acid levels that have built up over time have now formed sharp crystals that embed in your joints and soft tissues. This causes irritation to the joint, leading to inflammation.

Statistics show that 78% of sufferers experience a second attack within 6 months and up to 2 years later. Each subsequent attack tends to be worse in severity than the first and it spreads to more than one joint over time.

It is this stage that prompt treatment is highly necessary. The pain and flare may go away on its own, but can begin to damage your body. Some people have one flare and it doesn't return, but left untreated it may progress to chronic gout.

Stage 3: Interval Gout

During this stage, you may be out dancing the night away! The symptoms of gout have completely cleared up and you feel great. The bad news is, you still have gout as long and your uric acid levels are still elevated. They can remain elevated even during this "quiet" stage, and the crystals may still be present in your joints and soft tissues near the joints. It is quite possible for damage to your joints to continue, even when the gout is silent.

If you have a risk of recurrent flares, your doctor may have you continue on your gout treatment plan and/or medications even when gout is "silent."

Stage 4: Chronic Gout

With proper treatment and vigilance, hopefully you don't ever have to experience this stage of gout. After years of elevated uric acid levels, gout can cause you permanent disability. You may experience attacks closer together and they don't go away as quickly as earlier attacks. You may also begin to experience severe joint damage, kidney damage, or other severe complications. The time between your first attack and stage 4 is around 10 years.

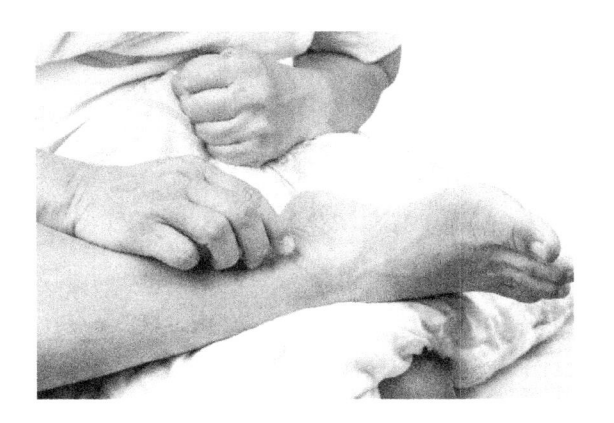

Causes of Gout

As we discussed before, gout is caused by elevated uric acid levels in your blood. This may lead you to the question, "where do we get uric acid from?"

A Breakdown of Cells

Quite simply put, uric acid is the breakdown of amino acids. Most of these come from animal proteins, but they are present in other foods and beverages. Not all amino acids turn to uric acid, but aminos that break down into purines turn into uric acid. Some beneficial amino acids are used by our body, and whatever is left over from purine amino acids form uric acid which is excreted by the kidneys.

While it may seem complicated, if we are healthy this process is quite normal and natural for our bodies to manage. Certain other factors can affect uric acid levels going up like, cancer. If you are on chemotherapy for cancer you can have excess uric acid because the chemo breaks down aminos in your body forming purines that turn into uric acid.

Most of the time, there are a lot of contributing factors to why uric acid levels rise and cause gout flares.

Underlying Disease and Medications

If you have underlying disease that affects your kidneys, you may not be able to clear uric acid from your body. There is also a genetic defect that affects the way you metabolize and get rid of uric acid, but this cause is actually rare and happens early in childhood.

Certain medications may increase your risk of gout. If you take diuretics that help pull fluids from your body, some may cause the uric acid to stay in your body. This is why it is important to let your doctor know if you are at risk if you are being prescribed new medications.

One very strong cause of gout is, diet. Since purines can cause uric acid levels to rise, a diet high in purines can lead to gout. Between 10% to 15% of our purines come from foods that we eat. Let's take a look at some of the foods that can cause gout.

Gout Causing Foods

Foods that can lead to or trigger gout are higher in purines than other foods. While you wouldn't want to cut certain things completely, you may need to talk to your doctor about the safe amounts you can consume to prevent your uric acid levels from getting too high. These foods include:

Foods High in Fat - Remember talking about "the disease of kings?" This was one reason that aristocracy was prone to gout in ancient days. They could afford the rich tasting and high fat meals. A high fat diet slows down the excretion of uric acid from the kidneys. The main culprits are:

Whole Milk Dairy Products
Stews and Soups with Stewed Meat
Gravies and Cream Sauces

Vegetables with Purines - You wouldn't normally think vegetables are bad for you, and they aren't really. Some vegetables do have large amounts of purines, but researchers are recommending you still eat them in moderation due to the other health benefits they can offer.

Animal Proteins – Animal proteins can be high in purines and send your uric acid levels through the roof if you overindulge. It is recommended that intake of animal proteins be limited to 3 ounces per serving and no more than 6 ounces daily.

In addition to the above, there are other dietary things that can raise your uric acid levels. Try to avoid:

1) Brewer's Yeast
2) Beer

When you drink alcoholic beverages, your body may produce high levels of purine compounds. It can also slow down uric acid excretion from your kidneys. This can cause your uric acid level to go up. Most doctors recommend that women limit alcohol to one alcoholic beverage daily and men need to limit alcoholic beverages to two drinks per day.

We will take a longer look at more dietary factors in the treatment section below. Now that we know high uric acid levels are the direct cause of gout, let's take a look at some of the lifestyle factors that can trigger a gout attack.

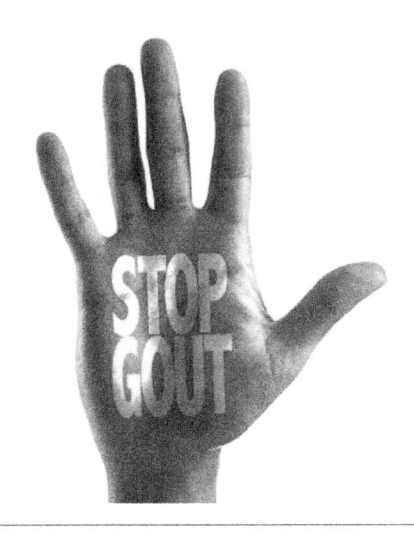

Lifestyle factors

Things you do every day don't necessarily cause gout, but they can be triggers. If you are overweight, use alcohol, and eat a rich diet you may be contributing to the risk of gout. Here are some of the lifestyle factors that may trigger a gout attack:

Medical or health triggers of gout

1) Physical stress on the body from illness or surgery

2) Injury to one or more joints

3) Diuretic use (water pills)

4) Certain medications like; aspirin, Levodopa for Parkinson's, Niacin, and Cyclosporine.

3) Chemotherapy for cancer

5) Infection in the body

Lifestyle triggers of gout

1) Diet high in purines

2) Excessive intake of alcohol

3) Crash dieting

4) Dehydration

5) Soft drinks high in sugar

If you are at risk for gout and have two or more of the above lifestyle factors, you need to watch closely for symptoms of gout. Prompt treatment and lifestyle changes can change the course of this condition for the better!

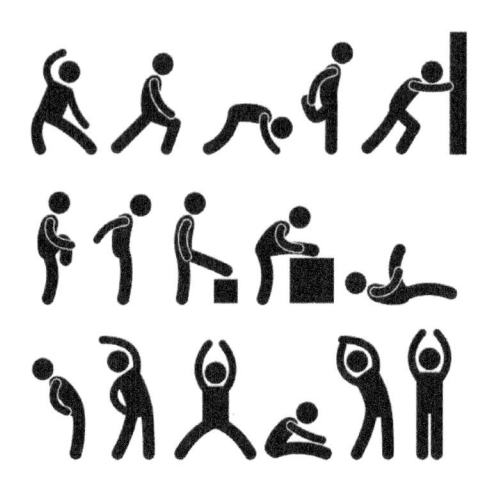

Symptoms of Gout

A first gout attack can be very scary with severe pain, redness and heat in the affected joint. You think back to what you might have done to injure yourself and can't remember anything that happened. You may however remember having an illness or another injury. The onset is very sudden and the symptoms at first may seem non-specific. The most confusing thing is that the first attack, you may only feel symptoms in one joint. Later attacks tend to affect more than one joint.

If symptoms are ignored and gout is not treated promptly you may have longer more severe attacks that spread to most of your joints. Gout can stick around and turn into chronic pain. If you develop tophi or uric acid crystals the joints may become damaged.

Preventing chronic gout is key. This way you can avoid some of the complications like kidney stones or other damage to your body. In order to make sure you get prompt treatment, watch out for these symptoms:

Pain in any joint. You may wake up from a sound sleep in excruciating pain in one joint. This is usually accompanied by swelling, heat, and redness. Most often it affects the joint in your large toe. It is most common during the night or first thing in the morning. People notice even the weight of the sheets hurt. When you get up, you may not even want to put your shoes on if your foot is affected.

Gout pain tends to peak 24 to 48 hours after you first feel it, then the pain remains constant, and subsides over the next few days.

Fever. It is possible to run fever with an acute gout attack. Fevers can often run very high and you may even have signs of a bacterial infection in your joint. If this happens, you need immediate medical attention. Doctors can take some fluid from your joint to check for bacteria present and treat you with antibiotics. This will also help the doctor know the difference between gout and another condition, septic arthritis.

Redness. The joint and skin may appear very red or even dark purple in color. The skin may also be very shiny and smooth looking. As your gout clears up, you may notice the skin itches and it may start to peel off.

Decreased range-of-motion. If your big toe is affected, you won't be able to "wiggle your toe." If your elbow is affected, you won't be able to bend your arm. You will find that trying to move an affected body part causes extreme and excruciating pain. The affected joints feel very stiff from swelling and inflammation.

Everyone is unique and one person may only have pain and swelling in one joint. There may be other people who experience high fever and pain in multiple joints. Some people may even only experience one or two attacks and never have another. Others may go on to develop chronic gout. It depends on your genetic makeup, how fast you treat the attack, and compliance to your treatment plan.

Note: If symptoms are ignored and left untreated, gout can become chronic. The attacks will happen in "flares" and become more frequent and more intense over time. This is another reason to know the symptoms of gout and watch for them.

Signs of Chronic Gout

1) Two or more attacks in one-year

2) Consistently high levels of uric acid >12 mg/dL

3) High uric acid in the urine

4) Kidney Stones

5) The appearance of Tophi. Lumps under your skin made of uric acid crystals.

6) Signs of joint damage

7) Chronic pain in one or more joints

The best way to prevent chronic gout or complications is to get medical treatment right away. If you wake up in the morning with severe pain in one or more joints, contact your doctor as soon as the office opens!

Next, we will explore how your doctor diagnoses gout.

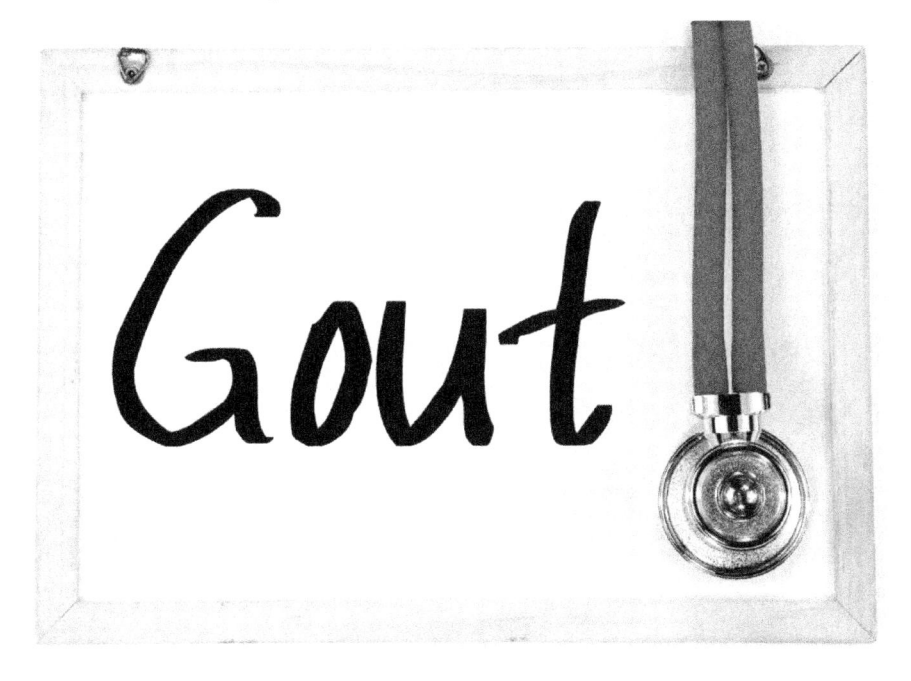

Diagnosing Gout

If you have symptoms of gout, get in to see your doctor right away. They will perform a battery of tests to see what is going on. There are other conditions that can cause these symptoms and those need to be ruled out before a diagnosis of gout can be confirmed. Tests include:

Blood Testing

You will most likely have the following blood tests:

Complete Blood Count (infection)

Uric Acid Levels (specific for gout *see note)

Kidney and Liver Function Tests

Tests for Rheumatoid Factor (rheumatoid arthritis)

Sedimentation Rate (inflammation levels)

24-hour Urine for Uric Acid

Note: Even though uric acid levels are widely used in gout diagnosis; these are not reliable. In around 10% of people having an acute gout attack, they have normal uric acid levels. Some people also have elevated uric acid levels, but do not have gout. It is also important to understand that uric acid levels may not be elevated during a gout flare. If you have a repeat flare of gout your doctor may re-check uric acid levels after the flare is over.

Other causes of elevated blood uric acid levels unrelated to gout:

Tumor Lysis Syndrome (cancer cells shedding into the bloodstream)

Psoriasis

Hypothyroidism (low thyroid hormone)

Kidney Disease

Chemotherapy

Aspiration of Affected Joint

This test is one of the most accurate tests for gout. This can rule out if the joint is infected or find the presence of uric acid crystals to confirm gout. The doctor takes a needle and inserts it into the joint that is affected. They will look at your joint fluid under a microscope for the uric acid crystals or bacteria. Aspiration can also find calcium crystals in the joint that can cause, pseudo gout. Pseudo gout is a condition like gout but not related.

Imaging Studies

The first acute attack of gout is essentially a soft tissue disease. Therefore, it is very hard to see the effects of gout on plain x-ray. There are other types of imaging that may be effective in diagnosing gout early on, but they are not routinely used since gout can often be confirmed with joint aspiration. Here is the breakdown of imaging studies that may be used:

X-Ray – The bony changes in gout usually do not show up on x-ray until around a year after the first attack. In some people, changes do not show up for 6 to 8 years after the initial attack. It just depends on how severe the disease is. This is why x-ray is an ineffective tool for diagnosing a first gout attack.

Ultrasound – There are new studies that show promise with using ultrasound
to diagnose gout. Uric acid crystals are very sensitive to ultrasound waves making
this test possibly very effective in diagnosing the first acute attack. In addition, ultrasound can pick up things x-ray can't such as; swelling in the tissues, increased joint fluid, and uric acid crystals.

CT Scan – CT scanning for gout tends to be a less reliable test for gout, but it may help
confirm diagnosis in a small number of patients that had normal uric acid levels from

aspirating a joint. This is because the uric acid crystals show up on CT and the doctor

can do a more localized joint aspiration guided by the CT scanner.

MRI – An MRI isn't usually a routine diagnostic test for gout because it can be very
expensive. It is a useful test if needed in the later stages of the disease to detect complications such as; joint damage, bone damage and the presence of tophi in tissues.

Once a diagnosis of gout is confirmed, medical treatment is started right away to reduce uric acid levels. A combination of medications, dietary and lifestyle changes can help reduce the length and severity of gout attacks. There are also several alternative therapies that can be a helpful addition to your treatment plan. Next, we will go over treatment options.

Medical Management of Gout

Medical management of gout is aimed at lowering uric acid levels in the body. This helps to reduce the severity and length of a flare. Treatment also helps reduce the risk of repeated flares over time.

Treatments for gout include; anti-inflammatory medications, uric acid lowering medications, dietary and lifestyle changes. Here are the most common treatments for gout:

Anti-inflammatory Medications

When gout pain sets in, narcotics and opioid medications may help temporarily, but actually do very little. Gout pain and inflammation needs medication that reduces inflammation and that in turn helps reduce the pain of the initial attack. These are given until gout medications have a chance to work on reducing the uric acid levels.

Anti-inflammatory medications that can help relieve pain and swelling with gout include:

Non-Steroidal Anti-inflammatory's (NSAID's)

A few of the NSAID's that are used in the treatment of gout include:

Ibuprofen

Indomethacin

Naproxen

Celecoxib

Meloxicam

Due to side-effects like; stomach upset, ulcers, thinning the blood, they are only used as long as needed and then stopped after the symptoms subside. In some circumstances, your doctor may find a safe anti-inflammatory that can be given long-term to prevent gout complications. In order to do this, you need to be free of things like; stomach bleeding, alcohol use, and stomach disease.

Corticosteroids

Corticosteroids like Prednisone can also be given for their anti-inflammatory action. They also help relieve pain. For milder cases, you may be given a prescription for oral corticosteroids. For more severe cases, you may be given a steroid injection in the affected joint.

These are only given as a last resort because they do have side-effects including; increased appetite, high blood sugar, high blood pressure, and mood swings. They can also lower the calcium in your bones.

Pain Relievers

Important Note: Aspirin should never be used with a gout attack. Aspirin can raise the uric acid levels in the blood. If you have to take aspirin for a chronic health condition, talk to your doctor. You may need a different medication during your gout flare.

Narcotics – Narcotics are only used if gout pain is severe. Narcotic pain medications often do not even work to manage gout pain. Gout pain is best managed by treating it at the source, uric acid. However, in the very early stages of a flare it can bring some relief.

Colchicine – If you are unable to take anti-inflammatory medications, colchicine is the drug of choice for gout pain relief. It works by lowering inflammation and swelling by blocking your white blood cells from rushing to the affected joint or joints. Side-effects include; nausea, vomiting, diarrhea, and abdominal pain.

Meds that lower uric acid levels

Your doctor will most likely prescribe medications to lower the levels of uric acid in your blood. You may even continue to take these after your acute flare to lower your risk of flares in the future. These medications slow down the amount of uric acid your body produces:

Allopurinol – Allopurinol is a long-term medication that helps keep uric acid levels low in the blood. It will help to reduce the severity or prevent future flares. Understand that if you are taking this medication and do have an acute flare, you may need to go back on one of the above anti-inflammatory medications. Side-effects include; Diarrhea, nausea, rash, sore throat, fever, and headache. Call your doctor if you develop red blistered or peeling skin.

Febuxostat – This drug is also known as, Uloric and is one of the newer gout medications. It works by blocking one of the enzymes that convert purines into uric acid in your body. There is a slight risk that as the medication works to break down uric acid crystals, you may have a gout flare. Side-effects include; rash, nausea, dizziness, and skin rash.

Probenecid – This drug lowers uric acid levels by increasing the amount you excrete from your kidneys. It is only used to prevent future gout attacks and will not treat an active gout flare. This medication does have side-effects including; kidney stones, abdominal pain, and rash.

Lesinurad – This is a new medication approved by the FDA in 2015. This medication works in conjunction with other gout medications to lower uric acid by increasing kidney excretion. Side-effects that have been reported are; flu-like symptoms, headache, stomach issues, and elevated creatinine levels. There is a warning that this drug should not be used by people at risk for kidney failure.

Pegloticase – This new medication became FDA approved in 2010. It is given by intravenous route and helps to lower uric acid in people who don't respond to other treatments. Side-effects include; gout flare, nausea, stuffy nose, bruising, and constipation.

Surgical Intervention

If gout is diagnosed and treated early, surgical intervention isn't normally necessary. If you don't get early treatment and gout progresses, it may warrant the need for surgery to remove any tophi that are causing issues with joint mobility or even circulation.

You may be referred to an orthopedic surgeon if your doctor finds too much damage to your; skin, cartilage, tendons, or bones. Inflammation may be hard to control and the tophi may have become embedded in the joint areas. Tophi can go quickly from a fluid filled cyst structure to a hard and chalk like lesion. These can cause pressure on your blood vessels, muscles and nerves near the joint. Surgeons may suggest removal if:

Tophi reduce the ability to use your tendons
Large unsightly tophi
Severe pain
Compression to blood vessels
Skin begins to die off (necrosis)
If the compression of blood vessels is severe, surgery will be strongly encouraged. This is important for older adults that have blockage of blood vessels in the lower limbs. There is a slight risk of amputation to a toe if gout is causing severe enough blood flow issues.

Keep in mind that with well managed gout, surgical intervention is actually uncommon.

Alternative Therapies for Gout

With your doctor's okay, there are alternative and complimentary therapies that may help reduce the severity of gout flares. Always make sure you let your doctor know if you are using alternative therapies. With herbal remedies, there can be drug interactions with gout medications. Some of them, your doctor may approve as complimentary therapy in your treatment plan. Never try to "self-treat" gout at home without seeing a doctor. This could lead to severe complications.

Here are a few of the most common complimentary and/or alternative therapies for gout:

MSM – Methylsulfonylmethane or MSM is a natural substance that is completely organic. It comes from the earth in the form of sulfur and is actually derived from rain. It helps detox our bodies and reduce inflammation. It is commonly used in conjunction with glucosamine, however there isn't any clinical evidence that glucosamine has any effect on gout.

Vitamin C – Vitamin C and foods that contain citric acid may help reduce uric acid levels, and may possible help break up uric acid crystals. It is recommended to increase vitamin C foods in the diet. The recommended daily allowance of vitamin C for gout is 500 mg to 1500 mg daily.

Omega 3 Fatty Acids – Omega 3 fatty acids can help lower the levels of inflammation in the body. They can also help protect your heart and blood vessels from gout damage. Try to eat 2 to 3 servings of cold water fatty fish weekly. The following foods are high in Omega 3 fatty acids; Salmon, white fish, cod liver oil, flaxseeds, and walnuts. Some canned fish is high in Omega 3 fatty acids, but also high in purines like; sardines, tuna, and canned mackerel. If you decide to use Omega 3 supplements, make sure you check with your doctor if you are taking blood thinners.

Tart Cherry – Many large studies have shown that tart cherries that are very dark red in color may help reduce uric acid in gout. Studies also show that they may also lower inflammatory markers in the body, reducing inflammation. The recommended intake for arthritis is around ½ pound of cherries daily, or you can use them to make cherry juice.

Turmeric – Xanthine oxidase is one of the enzymes that increases uric acid level production from purines. Turmeric may help inhibit xanthine oxidase and lower inflammatory levels in the body.

Cranberry – One of the side-effects of gout is a high risk of kidney stones. Cranberry helps flush out the urinary tract and may reduce the risk of developing kidney stones. It only takes around one to two 8 ounce servings daily to receive these benefits.

Devil's Claw – Devil's claw has been shown in small studies to help reduce inflammation and pain in conditions like gout. Just use caution if you are a diabetic or on blood thinners.

Bromelain – This is an enzyme found in pineapple. It doesn't really help gout when used alone, but when used with other natural gout supplements it helps increase their absorption and effectiveness. Supplements combined with Bromelain tend to have more anti-inflammatory and pain relief action.

Nettle Tea Compress – Using a nettle tea compress daily may help increase uric acid excretion from your kidneys and reduce levels of inflammation in your joints. Brew 1 tsp. in hot water and soak a cloth in the tea. Place on affected joints.

Belladonna – Belladonna is a homeopathic remedy that reduces heat in the body. It may reduce things like; hot burning pain, swelling, and restlessness due to pain.

Rhus toxicodendron – Another homeopathic remedy, Rhus can help relieve joints that are very stiff due to intense swelling. It may also lower arthritic pain in cold conditions.

Ledum – On the flipside of Rhus, Ledum works well for pain you feel when you are hot. If your joints are swollen with mottling, Ledum tends to work better.

Berberis vulgaris – Berberis vularis is homeopathic and helps to reduce pain spasms. It is most helpful for pain you feel when you walk. It is indicated if you are suffering from kidney stones and/or back pain.

Notes: When using vitamin supplements, try to avoid too much vitamin A or niacin. There are studies that show they may compete in the kidneys and lower uric acid excretion.

Regardless of the method of treatment you choose, your doctor will suggest that you make some dietary changes. Here is more info on a healthy diet for gout.

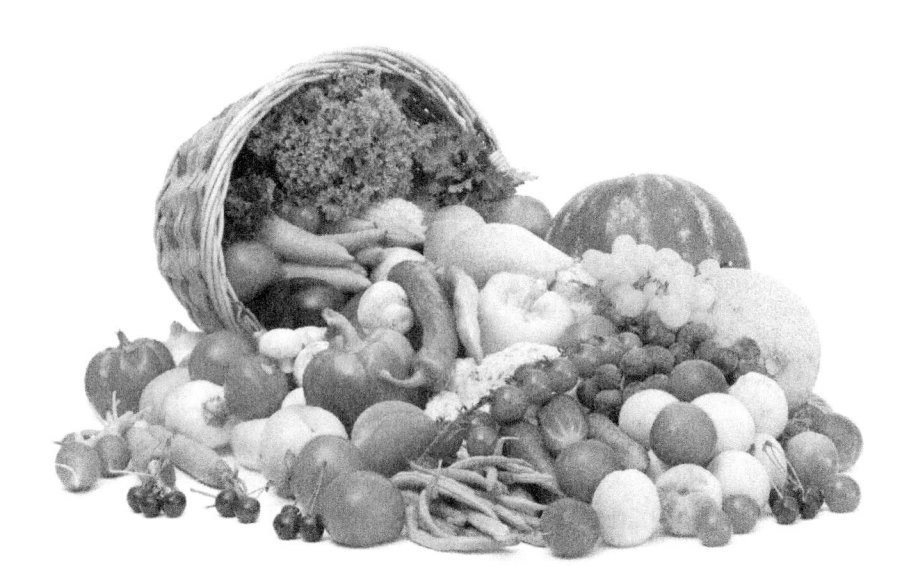

Gout Diet

For many years, doctors focused on all the things you shouldn't eat with gout. Gout treatment focused on avoiding foods that were high in purines. Most gout diets were boring and devoid of some very important nutrients. While it is important to adhere to a diet that helps you reduce the uric acid in your body to avoid uric acid crystals in your joints and soft tissues, new research has found certain foods that were once feared are now understood to be beneficial to gout when eaten in moderation.

The new developments in dietary management now recommend that a low-calorie diet is much more effective in lowering levels of uric acid in your body. While you still want to limit red meat and animal proteins, the focus is more on lowering your intake of refined sugar, carbohydrates, and processed food, and adding in fruits, vegetables, and low-fat dairy.

You will need to eat a healthy and balanced diet to keep your body healthy, lose weight, and control uric acid levels. Here is a quick rundown of foods you should eat and foods to avoid with gout:

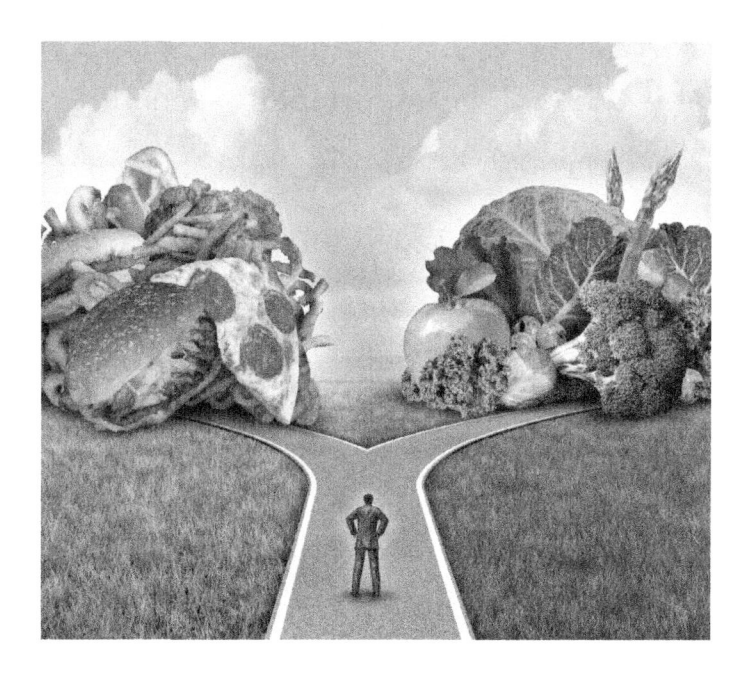

Foods to Avoid:

Avoid whole milk, whole milk yogurt, and whole milk cheeses.

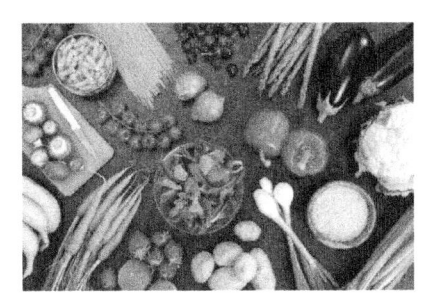

Vegetables

Your body needs vegetables as part of a balanced diet. Recent studies have changed the course of gout diets regarding vegetables. Doctor's used to recommend completely avoiding vegetables like; spinach, mushrooms, and asparagus. Good news, not anymore! It was found their content of purines isn't as high as once thought, plus these vegetables have other nutrients that are necessary to help reduce uric acid levels produced when you eat animal proteins. Just make sure you eat them in moderation.

Any other vegetables not mentioned above are in the free and clear. Go ahead, eat your veggies!

Foods to Avoid: Previously, gout sufferers were told to avoid beans and legumes. New studies have shown that despite their purine content, they are a better source of protein than meats when included in moderation in a gout diet.

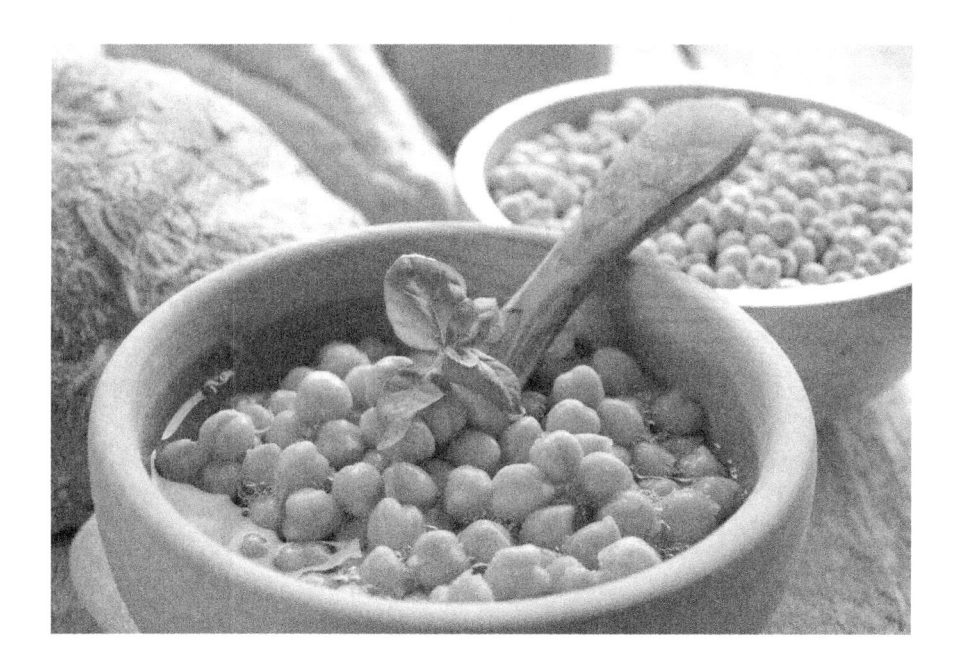

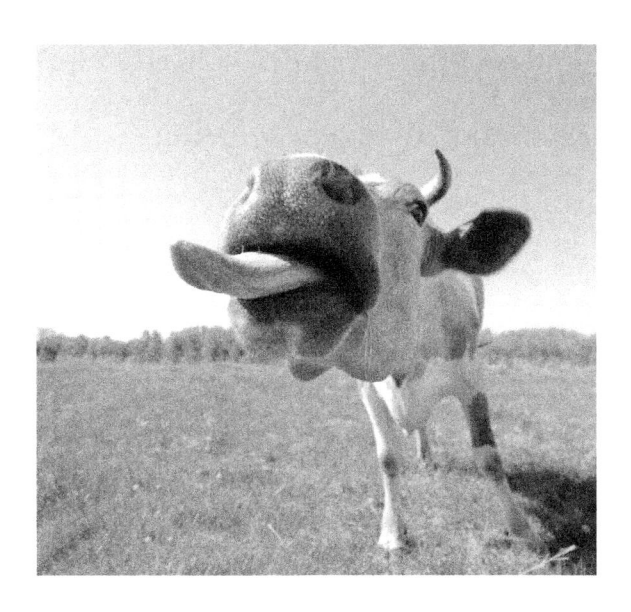

Animal Proteins

This is another area where recent studies have shown that animal proteins aren't as risky for gout sufferers as once thought. While they still want people at risk or suffering from gout to limit red meat and organ meat, you can eat up to 6 ounces of chicken, duck, ham, or pork. You can eat a 4 ounce serving of fish, beef, or shellfish.

Foods to Avoid: Bacon, organ meats (liver, brain, kidneys), anchovies, sardines, salmon, veal, and turkey. Reduce your intake of the following; soups made with stewed meats, gravies made with meat fat, and cream sauces.

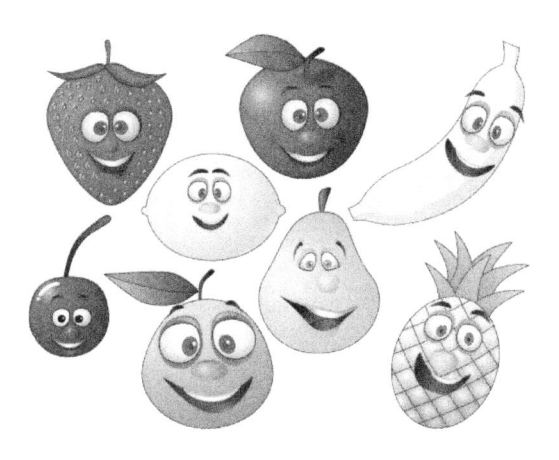

Fresh Fruits

Getting enough fiber in your diet with gout is really important. One of the ways to get enough fiber is to consume fruit that is high in fiber. These include; pears, bananas, and plums. They are also low purine fruits.

Another way to benefit your body with fruit is to choose the types that are high in flavonoids. These antioxidants help detox your body, lower inflammation, and even help clear uric acid. Fruit that is rich in flavonoids is red in color. The best fruits are; strawberries, raspberries, red grapes, and plums.

Foods to Avoid: Dried fruits. Dried fruits contain about 107 mg of purines and can make up to 100 mg of uric acid in your body. Ask your doctor or dietician, but you may need to limit things like raisins or dates. Use caution because they may be hidden in some baked goods.

Other Foods to Avoid

Raisins

Sunflower Seeds

Caviar

Coffee Intake

Coffee has been on the radar lately for numerous health benefits. Now researchers have found that it may help reduce the risk of gout, reduce uric acid levels in gout sufferers, and may reduce the frequency of gout flares. One study was very large and included over 45,000 men who drank four to five cups of coffee daily. Their risk of gout was 40 percent lower than men who did drink coffee. The numbers actually got better for men who drank six or more cups of coffee daily. Their risk of gout was lowered by 59 percent!

If you have high blood pressure or sensitivity to caffeine, discuss increasing your coffee intake with your doctor. It could do more harm than good. The good news is, decaf coffee was found to have a mild effect in gout prevention, although less than caffeinated coffee it did help some.

Increased Water Intake

Last but not least, if you have gout you have to increase your water intake. Increasing water can help reduce the amount of gout flares that you have. The studies done on water and gout show that people who drank at least five to eight glasses of water the day before a gout flare had up to a 40 percent lower risk of gout flares than people who drank one glass of water the day before. Gout flares can appear suddenly so you never know when they will hit. Your doctor can give you the best recommendation for how much water you need to be drinking every day.

Lifestyle Changes for Gout

Gout can be a manageable condition and future flares can be minimized or even prevented by making some simple changes to your lifestyle. It can be as easy as going for a walk after dinner, cutting back to one beer a day, and doing things to relieve stress in your life. Studies show that people tend to be more compliant with lifestyle changes if they are gradual and easy to handle.

These lifestyle changes can help you manage your gout and still enjoy a good quality of life:

Lower Your Alcohol Intake. The news on alcohol and gout hasn't changed. Especially with beer. Not only is alcohol dehydrating to your body, but hard liquor and beer can elevate uric acid levels in your blood. New studies show that it is probably a good idea to avoid beer and hard liquor, but there are no adverse effects with up to two glasses of wine a day.

Try Losing Weight. Losing weight can benefit your overall health. It can help prevent diabetes, high blood pressure, heart disease, and gout attacks. It is recommended that you try to keep your BMI as lower than 25. Waist size is also a very important factor. If you are female, your waist size needs to fall below 35 inches. Waist size should be below 40 inches for males. This can be done by following portion control, eating the right foods, and exercise.

Exercise. Now is a good time to add an exercise routine into your life. Exercising is good for your health and can keep gout under control. It can also be stress relieving. You will want to wait to start exercising until your gout flare has cleared. Always start with gentle stretches first to prevent strain. A good first exercise for joint pain sufferers is swimming. Other low-impact exercises are; slow walking, yoga, stationary bike, rowing, and tai chi. Remember to check with your doctor before starting exercise.

Reduce Stress. Both physical and emotional stress can increase the risk of gout flares. When you are sick, tired, or stressed your uric acid levels can rise. If you are physically ill or tired, let your doctor know so you can work to prevent a flare. If you are under high levels of emotional stress, try to do some stress relieving techniques. These include; exercise, meditation, journaling, and talking to someone about your feelings.

Rest Your Body. Your body needs enough rest to heal from gout. If you are experiencing pain, you need to rest the joints that are affected. Try to get at least 6 to 8 hours of sleep every night. This will help reduce the physical stress on your body and may even help prevent future flares.

Know The Signs of a Flare. Knowing the signs of a gout flare will help you catch things early and step up your game. While you won't be able to completely stop a flare, you can reduce the effects and maybe even minimize the severity. Even when you don't have symptoms, your uric acid level can be going up without you knowing it. The uric acid crystals may silently form over months and then one morning you wake up, and you are under attack.

Warning signs of subsequent gout attacks include:

Burning near an affected joint
Skin itching
Skin tingles
Joint stiffness
Soreness

Just like the first attack, you may not even know until you wake up with a stiff, sore, and swollen joint. If you do have signs of an impending flare, start your "home-care" routine right away. If your doctor gave you medication, give your doctor a call and you may be directed to start taking medication right away.

Complications of Gout

Chronic gout can lead to complications if not managed properly. Gout attacks are initially disabling. If you are working with your doctor and using a good treatment plan, your risk of complications can be lowered immensely. If you don't treat gout it can become chronic and cause injury to the joints, kidneys, and even your heart. Below are some of the complications of untreated or poorly treated gout:

Joint Damage and Disability

If uric acid levels remain high, uric acid crystals form in the soft tissues near your joints and even inside the joint. This causes damage to the cartilage and eventually breaks down the bone. Your joints will lose their shape and you will lose range-of-motion or ability to bend it. The tophi can grow very large and completely destroy your joint. This can lead to permanent inability to use the affected joint or joints and disability. Your joints can also become grossly disfigured.

Chronic Pain

In gout flares, the pain subsides over a one or two-week time period. Over time, untreated gout can lead to flares of pain that last longer and longer. Once joint damage begins to occur, pain flares can turn into chronic pain that does not go away. Chronic gout pain is very hard to treat because the only way to eliminate it is to remove the source, uric acid crystals.

Kidney Diseases

High uric acid levels in your blood passes through your kidneys to be filtered out. At first, this isn't usually a problem and increased water will help dilute the uric acid. If levels continue to be high in the urine, the uric acid mixes with other solids and forms kidney stones. This can become a chronic problem with chronic gout. Not to mention, uncomfortable.

Uric acid flowing through the kidneys over a long period of time can cause damage to the kidneys themselves. Chronic gout increases the risk for kidney disease. This can ultimately end in kidney failure if left untreated.

Heart Disease

There is a higher incidence of gout in people that have blood vessel issues like; high blood pressure, high triglycerides, and abdominal fat. The connection isn't completely understood, but gout is considered a factor that increases the risk of heart disease. The connection is even stronger in people who suffer from metabolic syndrome or low insulin sensitivity. If you have any of these conditions, you will need to work even more closely with your doctor to keep them under control if you develop gout.

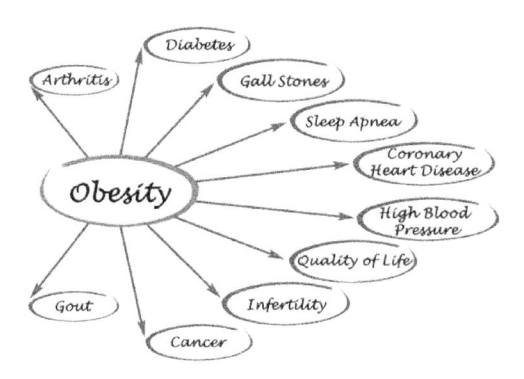

Obesity is connected to: Arthritis, Diabetes, Gall Stones, Sleep Apnea, Coronary Heart Disease, High Blood Pressure, Quality of Life, Infertility, Cancer, Gout.

Eye Problems

Chronic gout can lead to formation of uric acid crystals or tophi in the eyes. This can lead to hemorrhaging in the eyes, increased eye pressure, cataracts, and dry eyes. If you suffer from gout, it is important to see an ophthalmologist to evaluate your eyes and treat any complications. One severe eye complication is, scleritis. If tophi form in the white part of your eye it can become inflamed. Scleritis is treated with steroid or anti-inflammatory eye drops. If left untreated, this can lead to blindness.

Lung Disease

Gout associated lung disease is a rare complication, and can happen early in the disease if uric acid levels are not lowered quickly. Tophi can form inside the lungs causing shortness of breath, cough, and even respiratory failure. It can lead to death if left untreated.

Long Term Prognosis

The long-term prognosis for gout has never been better if treated promptly and properly. New research, new medications, and new dietary guidelines can help preserve your health. You may notice that when you begin treatment, your gout may be a little more frequent and severe. Patients often quit treatment due to this effect. It is important to remember that continuing to take your gout medications will prevent complications and chronic disease.

One risk of death from gout is due to cardiac complications. One study suggested that untreated gout with moderately high levels of uric acid can increase risk of cardiovascular disease by 42% and risk of cardiac death by 58%. The higher the uric acid levels the higher the risk of death. If uric acid levels are extremely high, the risk of death from gout goes up to 77% if untreated and risk of death from cardiac complications goes up to 209% in untreated gout.

Prevention Strategy

With all the recent developments in gout management, it has truly become a manageable condition. Thirty, Forty, and even Fifty years ago gout was a very high risk to health and life from complications. If you work with your doctor, you can devise a treatment plan that easily fits into your routine.

Gout pain is one of the most severe arthritic pains there is. Unfortunately, narcotic and opioid pain medications are often only effective temporarily. It is one pain that you definitely don't want coming back time and time again. Remember, the only way to control gout pain is lowering uric acid levels.

When you are not having an acute flare, you will still need to stick to your gout diet, exercise routine, and possibly medications. This will hopefully spare you from ever feeling that horrid pain ever again!

If you are not yet a gout sufferer and are at risk, the one way you can reduce the risk of gout attacks is to come up with a long-term strategy for prevention.

If you are found to have high uric acid levels in your blood for any reason, your doctor will need a medical history from you and your family. A family history of gout and other risk factors may increase your risk of an acute gout attack.

When your blood levels are elevated, your doctor may decide to check uric acid levels in your urine. This is a 24-hour test that you deposit all of your urine into a large lab container. They will check the amount of uric acid you excrete in a 24-hour period. Some people have naturally high levels of uric acid. This doesn't always lead to a gout flare or issues, but your doctor may want to treat you with medication to prevent a gout attack.

Sometimes, people at risk for an acute gout attack will be put on a very small dose of anti-inflammatory medication for prevention. These may be used in combination with other gout medications.

This method of prevention is used for both people at risk for gout or people who have had more than two gout flares. The criteria include:

One or two very severe attacks

Any evidence of joint damage

Kidney Stones that contain uric acid crystals

Risk of developing tophi (uric acid crystals) in soft tissues

Congenital hyperuricemia (from birth)

Kidney disease with elevated uric acid

People with these increased risks will most likely be placed on what they call a, **Uricosuric** medication to help your kidneys flush more uric acid from your body. Another reason these drugs may be used is if you have high uric acid levels in your blood, but low levels in your 24-hour urine test. If you have the above risks meet the criteria for this method of gout prevention if:

You are not at risk for kidney disease

You do not have or have had kidney stones

You are eating a normal diet

You are less than age 60

You do not have tophi (uric acid crystal formation)

In patients who are older and do not meet the above criteria, doctors may use low dose **allopurinol** to stop increased uric acid production in the body. It has been found safe to use long-term in the elderly, but can cause a gout attack in the beginning of treatment. This is why anti-inflammatory medications are used in the beginning of treatment. The good news about this medication is it can help reduce high cholesterol levels and reduce the risk of cardiac complications.

Coming up with a good prevention strategy now if you have a family history of gout or if you have a history of gout can save your health. Have uric acid levels checked before symptoms appear and if they are elevated, work with your doctor on a diet plan and make lifestyle changes now. It is possible to be at risk for gout, have elevated uric acid levels, and ward off an attack or future attacks. It just takes perseverance and commitment to your health. Latest research has developed new medications that can be taken long-term to prevent future gout attacks from occurring.

Summary of Latest Gout Research

This section will summarize any latest developments in gout research. The scientific community is constantly advancing in gout research. Gout treatments keep getting better and there are fewer complications from gout if you follow the treatment plan you and your doctor create.

The new findings on gout are:

Insulin Sensitivity/Metabolic Syndrome – As stated above, one of the related factors in gout is metabolic syndrome and insulin sensitivity. Researchers found that when limiting protein foods in the diet, patients took in too many carbohydrates. This led to an increase in the levels of insulin in the body and reduced sensitivity to insulin. This actually complicated gout.

It is now known that a low-fat and low carbohydrate diet can actually lower insulin levels in your body and subsequently reduce uric acid levels. It was also found that lowering saturated fat in the diet helps decrease insulin secretion.

Beans/Legumes – Beans and legumes were once regarded as unhealthy foods for gout due to high purine levels. Researchers have found that replacing animal proteins with plant proteins actually help lower uric acid levels even if they do contain purines. They are also recommending increasing intake of nuts to help supplement plant based proteins.

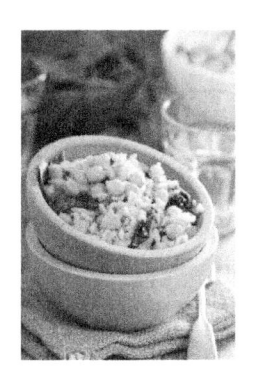

Coffee Intake – The new recommendations calls for two to three cups of coffee daily to help reduce uric acid in the body. Research showed that regular caffeinated coffee reduced the levels the most, but if caffeine is contraindicated, decaffeinated coffee still has some effect. It is not recommended to drink too much coffee, and you should use caution if you have issues with kidney stones. Coffee can be dehydrating so make sure you take in adequate water. The study showed no effects on uric acid from drinking tea.

Dairy – New research shows that low-fat dairy can reduce uric acid levels. Whole milk products are not advised and can raise uric acid levels. The new recommendation is gout sufferers get two servings of low-fat dairy products each day. This also helps weight loss efforts and prevention of osteoporosis.

Fructose/Fruit Sugars – Fructose and high fructose corn syrup used to sweeten drinks and food can raise uric acid levels very high. This has been found to be one of the huge risk factors for gout. Researchers recommend avoiding products that are sweetened with fructose or high fructose corn syrup.

In addition, if you drink beverages sweetened with fructose cold, the increase in uric acid is even higher. This may be because of warmer weather when you increase your intake of cold beverages. In warmer months, try to switch to unsweetened cold beverages and avoid any cold beverages containing fructose. Excessive intake of cold beverages containing fructose also contributes to weight gain.

Alcohol – Research is ongoing on which alcoholic drinks have more purines. Any type of alcohol lowers the amount of uric acid your kidneys can filter out and excrete. It is reported that beer and hard liquor have the most purines, but it is safe to drink one to two glasses of wine daily. Researchers are now finding that all types of alcohol may have the same effect on uric acid excretion. The new recommendations are to either quit drinking completely with gout or have no more than one drink daily.

BMI – Men who have a BMI over 27.5 have a 16-fold higher risk of a gout attack than men in the BMI range of 20 to 25.

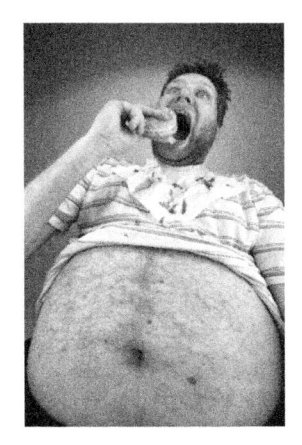

Exercise – It is understandable that exercise during a gout flare is impossible. You may even be scared to exercise after the flare has ended. New research shows that people with gout that do a moderate amount of cardio exercise have significantly lower levels of uric acid. Researchers are still looking at how exercise plays out with gout. What they have found is that uric acid excretion peaks during cardio exercise, but then almost stops as the body recovers from cardio and can actually raise uric acid levels. This may cause symptoms to become worse after exercise. Moderate exercise still has benefits like; losing weight and increased insulin sensitivity. Check with your doctor to see what exercise is best for you.

These new findings make following a gout treatment plan easier than ever. All it takes is eating a healthy balanced diet, avoiding high fructose foods, and adding low-fat dairy. Couple that with a plan to lose excess weight, medications, and some exercise for success!

Closing

There are far better ways to live like royalty than living with gout flares. If you do develop an acute gout attack, there are plenty of new treatments and recommendations to help ease your symptoms and prevent future flares.

Gout diets don't have to be boring and devoid of delicious foods either. The new dietary recommendations give you back foods that were once forbidden. As long as you practice moderation and eat a wide variety of healthy foods, you can manage gout even better now.

It seems researchers are still "on the fence" about alcohol intake. To drink wine or not to drink wine. Better to follow the guidelines as they stand and just not overdo it. One to two drinks a day may still be just fine with your doctors okay.

Medications for gout are getting better and better. There are new combination therapies that are proving to be very effective in controlling and reducing gout flares.

The best news is; gout can be managed and you can have a good quality of life!

Thank you for your readership, and I hope this can help. My gout flair ups remain under control, with a consistent healthy diet, and exercise. I do hope the same for everyone else as well. If you find time, please do review this book, and let others know your knowledge on the subject. Maybe you have great natural remedies that you have learned, that can help others. We are all students of life. And your knowledge can help someone who may not yet know what you do.

Thank you

Steven

References

AARON T. EGGEBEEN, M. (2007). University of Pittsburgh Athritis Institute. *American Family Physician*, 801-808.

Choi HK1, C. G., & Rheum., A. (2007). Coffee, Tea, and Caffeine Consumption and Serum Uric Acid Level. *National Health and Nutrition Examination Survey*, 816-821.

Grassi W, O. T. (2015). Use of Ultrasound for Diagnosis and Monitoring of Outcomes in Crystal Arthropathies. *Current Opinion in Rheumatology*, 147-155.

Jasvinder A. Singh, S. G. (2011). Current Opinion Rheumatology. *10.1097/BOR.0b012e3283438e13*, 192-202.

Jing Lin, G.-Q. Z.-Y.-S.-G. (2013). Characteristics of Ocular Abnormalities in Gout Patients. *International Journal of Opthamology*, 307-311.

LARMON, W. A., & KURTZ, J. F. (1958). The Surgical Management of Chronic Tophaceous Gout. *Journal of Bone and Joint Surgery*, 743-772.

Lombard, M. (2010). Krause's Food, Nutrition, & Diet Therapy. *The Specialist Forum*, 60-64.

Robert G. Smith, D. M. (2009). The Diagnosis and Treatment of Gout. *US Pharmacist*, 40-47.

Rymal, E. (2014). Journal of the American Academy of Physician Assistants. *doi: 10.1097/01.AA.0000453233.24754.ec*, 26-31.

University of Maryland Medical Center. (2016, April 1). *Gout*. Retrieved from University of Maryland Medical Center: http://umm.edu/health/medical/altmed/condition/gout

Vidula Bhole, M. d. (2010). Arthritis & Rheumatism. *Vol. 62, No. 4*, 1069-1076.

Yuan-Sheng Zang1, Z. F. (2012). Gout Associated Lung Disease. *Rheumatology. Oxford Journal*, ker354.

Yuqing Zhang, 1. T. (2013). Cherry Consumption and the Risk of Recurrent Gout Attacks. *Arthritis Rheumatology*.

We would like to leave you with some extra bonus material. Here are some delicious smoothie recipes that help with inflammation in the body.

These recipes are taken from these two books. Check them out on Amazon.

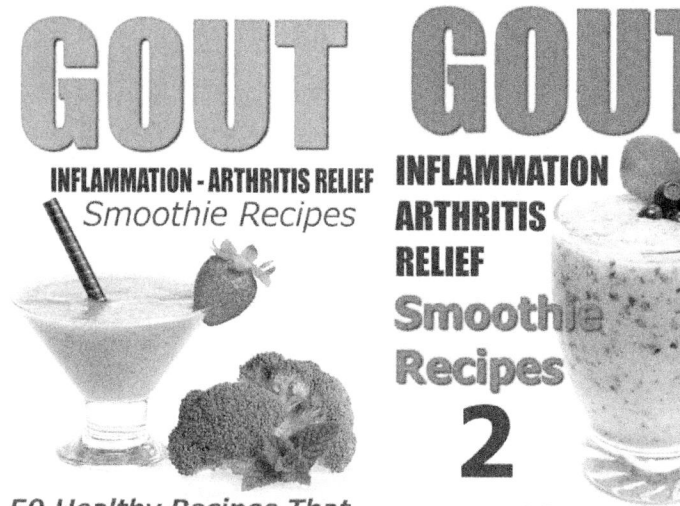

Apple Pie: Apple, Cinnamon, Almond

Servings: 2

Ingredients

- 2 apples, cored and quartered, with skin
- 2 tbsp. creamy almond butter
- 1 cup original almond milk, unsweetened
- ½ cup low-fat plain yogurt
- ½ tsp. cinnamon
- ¼ tsp. nutmeg
- Pinch cloves
- Pinch of ginger

Directions

1. Combine ingredients in a blender. Cover and blend until smooth.

Nutritional Information (per serving)

- Calories 224.7
- Fat 10.6 g
- Carbohydrates 25.9 g
- Sugar 17.2 g
- Protein 10.1 g

Beet the Rush Smoothie: Beet, Strawberry, Raspberry

Servings: 2
Ingredients
- 1 small beetroot, trimmed and quartered
- 1 cup frozen strawberries, unsweetened
- 1 small banana, peeled
- ½ cup red raspberries
- ¾ cup orange juice

Directions
1. Preheat oven to 400° F.
2. While oven is preheating, wash and trim leaves off of beet. Cut into quarters and place on a baking sheet. Bake for 30 minutes, or until soft.
3. Combine ingredients in a blender. Cover and blend until smooth.

Nutritional Information (per serving)
- Calories 146.2
- Fat .8 g
- Carbohydrates 35.5 g
- Sugar 14.4 g
- Protein 2.5 g

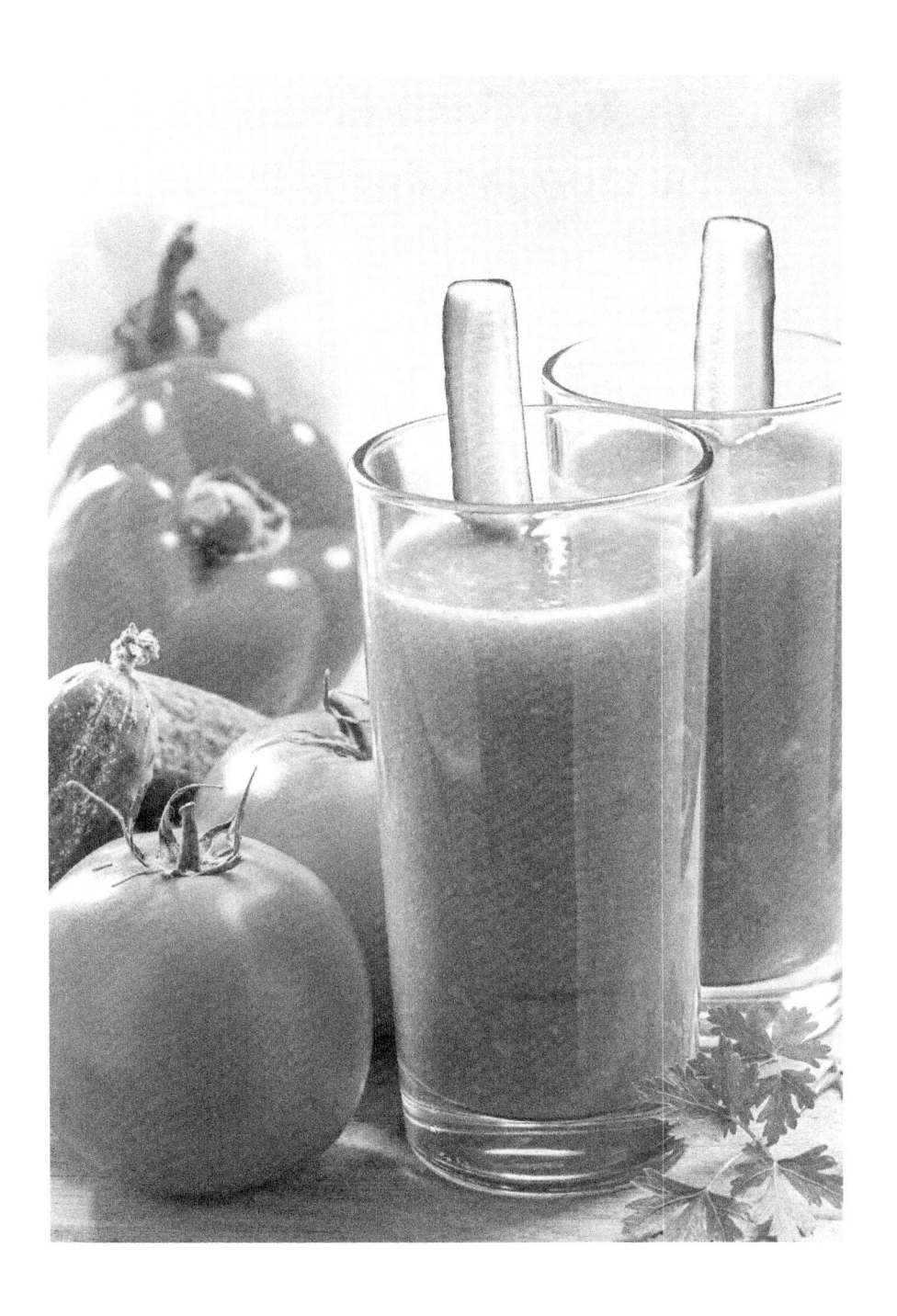

Watermelon-Basil Lemonade: Watermelon, Strawberry, Basil

Servings: 2
Ingredients
- 5 cups watermelon, cubed and seeded
- 1 cup frozen strawberries, unsweetened
- ½ cup cucumber slices
- ½ cup lemon juice
- 4 fresh basil leaves

Directions
1. Combine ingredients in a blender. Cover and blend until smooth.

Nutritional Information (per serving)
- Calories 164.2
- Fat 2 g
- Carbohydrates 39 g
- Sugar 28.4 g
- Protein 3.3 g

Creamy Cantaloupe: Cantaloupe, Pineapple, Banana

Servings: 2
Ingredients
- 1 cup cantaloupe chunks
- ½ cup frozen pineapple chunks, unsweetened
- ½ banana, peeled
- ¼ cup shredded carrots
- ½ cup coconut water

Directions
1. Combine ingredients in a blender. Cover and blend until smooth.

Nutritional Information (per serving)
- Calories 102
- Fat 0 g
- Carbohydrates 25 g
- Sugar 19 g
- Protein 2 g

Peary-Cherry: Pear, Cherry

Servings: 2
Ingredients
- 1 pear, cored and chopped, with skin
- 1 small apple, cored and quartered, with skin
- 1 cup frozen cherries, pitted
- ½ cup beet juice*
- ½ almond milk, original unsweetened
- 3-5 ice cubes

Substitute with cherry or apple juice, if desired.

Directions
1. Combine ingredients in a blender. Cover and blend until smooth.

Nutritional Information (per serving)
- Calories 135.3
- Fat .8 g
- Carbohydrates 33.1 g
- Sugar 21.4 g
- Protein 1.6 g

Peaches and Green: Peach & Avocado

Servings: 2
Ingredients
- 2 ripe peaches, pitted and quartered
- 1 ripe avocado, pitted and peeled
- 1 cup vanilla almond milk, unsweetened
- ½ small banana, peeled
- 1 tbsp. creamy cashew butter*

Substitute with almond or peanut butter, if desired.

Directions
1. Combine ingredients in a blender. Cover and blend until smooth.

Nutritional Information (per serving)
- Calories 250.2
- Fat 17.1 g
- Carbohydrates 26 g
- Sugar 12.3 g
- Protein 4.9 g

Sweet Potato Pie: Sweet potato & Banana

Servings: 2
Ingredients
- 1 medium sweet potato
- ½ banana, peeled
- 1 cup vanilla almond milk, unsweetened
- 2 tbsp. creamy cashew butter*
- ½ tsp. cinnamon
- Pinch of nutmeg
- Pinch of ginger
- Pinch of allspice
- 3-4 ice cubes

Substitute with peanut or almond butter, if desired.

Directions
1. Preheat oven to 350°F.
2. While oven is preheating, wash the potato. Pierce several times with a fork before baking it in the oven for 50 minutes, or until tender. Remove peel from potato and cool.
3. Once cooled, combine ingredients in a blender. Cover and blend until smooth.

Nutritional Information (per serving)
- Calories 179.8
- Fat 9.2 g
- Carbohydrates 21.7 g
- Sugar 6.2 g
- Protein 4.7 g

Sweet Peach Tea: Peach, Green Tea

Servings: 2
Ingredients
- 2 ripe peaches, pitted
  - 1 cup water
  - 1 green tea packet*
  - 2 dates, pitted
- 1 small apple, cored and quartered, with skin
  - 3-4 ice cubes

Substitute with peach tea, if desired.

Directions
1. Bring 1 cup water to boil, then let cool for approximately 2 minutes, or until 175°F. Steep one green tea packet in water for 1 minute. Remove packet and let cool.
2. Combine ingredients in a blender. Cover and blend until smooth.

Nutritional Information (per serving)
- Calories 139.7
  - Fat .3 g
- Carbohydrates 36.2 g
  - Sugar 29.1 g
  - Protein 1.3 g

Sparkling Peach Spritzer: Peach, Grape

Servings: 2
Ingredients
- ½ cup apple juice
- 1 tbsp. lime juice
- 1 ripe peach, pitted and quartered
- 1 cup seedless green grapes
- 4-5 ice cubes

Directions
1. Combine ingredients in a blender. Cover and blend until smooth

Nutritional Information (per serving)
- Calories 107
- Fat .3 g
- Carbohydrates 27.8 g
- Sugar 16.3 g
- Protein 1 g

Cherry Citrus Smoothie: Pineapple, Cherry

Servings: 2

Ingredients

- 1 cup frozen pineapple chunks, unsweetened
- 1 cup cherries, pitted
- ½ cup orange juice
- ½ cup coconut water

Directions

1. Combine ingredients in a blender. Cover and blend until smooth.

Nutritional Information (per serving)

- Calories 157
- Fat 0 g
- Carbohydrates 37 g
- Sugar 29 g
- Protein 3 g

Sunrise Smoothie: Kiwi, Watermelon, Strawberry

Servings: 2

Ingredients

- 1 cup watermelon chunks, seedless
- 1 kiwi, peeled and sliced
- ½ cup strawberries, halved
- ½ cup original almond milk, unsweetened
- 4-5 ice cubes

Directions

1. Combine ingredients in a blender. Cover and blend until smooth.

Nutritional Information (per serving)

- Calories 64.8
- Fat 1 g
- Carbohydrates 14.6 g
- Sugar 6.7 g
- Protein 1.3 g

Better Birthday Cake: Vanilla, Spinach, Banana

Servings: 2
Ingredients
- ½ banana, peeled
- 1 banana, frozen
- 2 tbsp. creamy cashew butter*
- 1 cup vanilla almond milk, unsweetened
- ½ tsp. pure vanilla extract
- 2 cups spinach

*Substitute with almond butter, if desired.

Directions
1. Combine ingredients in a blender. Cover and blend until smooth.

Nutritional Information (per serving)
- Calories 214.6
- Fat 9.4 g
- Carbohydrates 30.5 g
- Sugar 16.5 g
- Protein 5.1 g

Blue Raspberry Tea: Blueberry, Raspberry, White Tea

Servings: 2
Ingredients
- 1 cup low-fat blueberry yogurt
- 1 tsp. lemon juice
- 1 cup red raspberries
- 1 cup blueberries
- 1 cup water
- 1 white tea bag
- 3-4 ice cubes

Directions
1. Bring 1 cup water to boil, then let cool for approximately 2 minutes, or until 175°F. Steep one white tea packet in water for 1 minute. Remove packet and let cool.
2. Combine ingredients in a blender. Cover and blend until smooth

Nutritional Information (per serving)
- Calories 120.7
- Fat .3 g
- Carbohydrates 27.4 g
- Sugar 14.4 g
- Protein 4.2 g

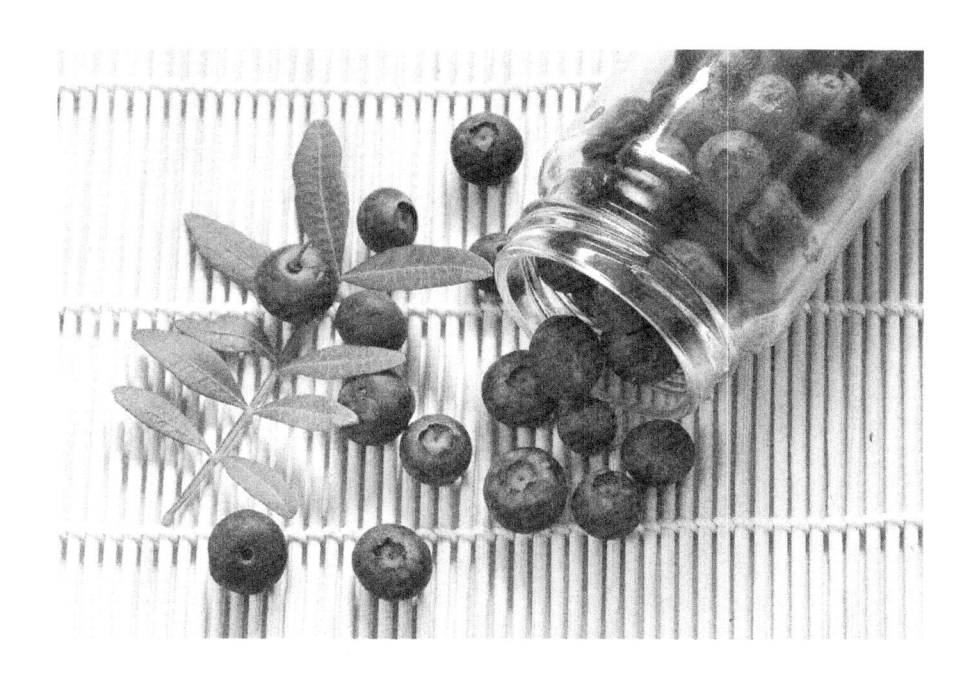

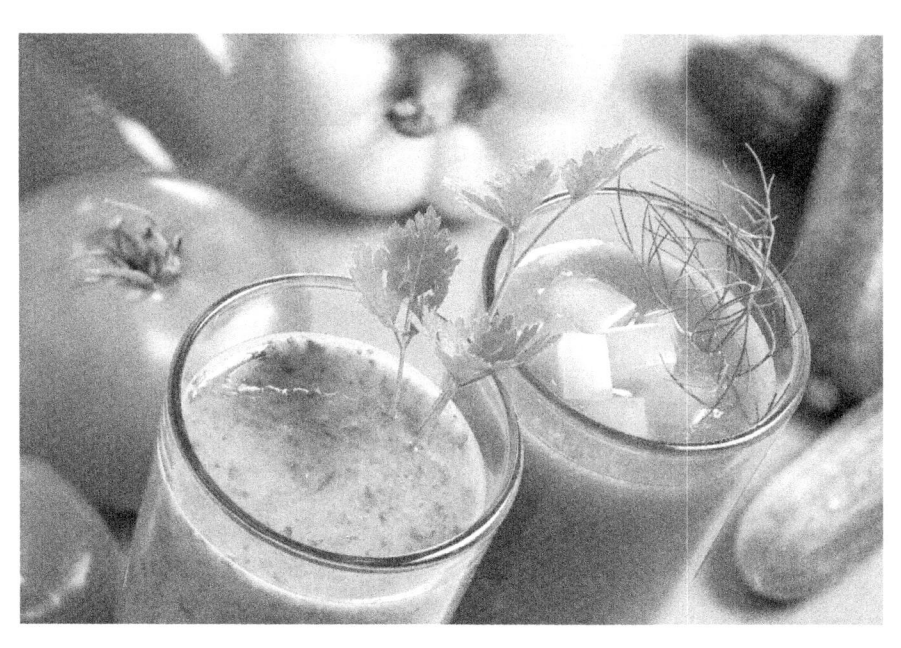

Blackberry Mango Tango: Blackberry, Mango, Honeydew

Servings: 2
Ingredients
- 1 cups frozen mango chunks
- 1 cup blackberries
- 1 cup honeydew melon chunks
- 1 cup coconut water
- 1 tsp. pure vanilla extract

Directions
1. Combine ingredients in a blender. Cover and blend until smooth.

Nutritional Information (per serving)
- Calories 108
- Fat 1 g
- Carbohydrates 25 g
- Sugar 16 g
- Protein 2 g

Mango Berry Smoothie: Mango, Blueberry

Servings: 2
Ingredients
- 1 cup blueberries
- 1 cup frozen mango chunks
- 1 cup original almond milk, unsweetened
- 1 tsp lemon juice
- 1 tbsp. raw coconut butter*
- 4-6 ice cubes

Substitute with almond butter, if desired.

Directions
1. Combine ingredients in a blender. Cover and blend until smooth.

Nutritional Information (per serving)
- Calories 155
- Fat 7 g
- Carbohydrates 24 g
- Sugar 17 g
- Protein 2 g

You've Broc-To Be Kidding: Broccoli, Blueberry, Orange

Servings: 2

Ingredients

- ¾ cup broccoli florets, de-stemmed
- 2 cups water
- 1 cup blueberries
- 1 orange, peeled and separated
- 1 cup orange juice
- 3-4 ice cubes

Directions

1. In a medium sauce pan, bring water to a boil. Boil broccoli for 7 minutes, or until tender. Remove from heat, drain, and let cool.
2. Combine ingredients in a blender. Cover and blend until smooth.

Nutritional Information (per serving)

- Calories 146.7
- Fat .6 g
- Carbohydrates 34.6 g
- Sugar 25.5 g
- Protein 3.5 g

Blackberry Cobbler: Blackberry, Almond

Servings: 2
Ingredients
- 1 ½ cups blackberries
- ½ cup original almond milk, unsweetened
- 2 tbsp. creamy almond butter
- ½ cup low-fat vanilla yogurt
- 1 tsp. cinnamon
- 1 tsp. vanilla extract
- 4-6 ice cubes
- Optional: add 1 Tbsp. raw honey for a sweeter smoothie

Directions
1. Combine ingredients in a blender. Cover and blend until smooth.

Nutritional Information (per serving)
- Calories 166.9
- Fat 9.1 g
- Carbohydrates 20.1 g
- Sugar 10.1 g
- Protein 4.3 g

Tasty and Refreshing Pineapple Avocado Smoothie

Total Time: 5 minutes

Serves: 4

Ingredients:

- 2 cups pineapple, cut into chunks
- 2 avocados, remove seed and scoop out
- 1 cup almond milk
- 1 large banana
- 2 cups chopped spinach
- 1 cup pineapple juice

Directions:

1. Add all ingredients into the blender and blend until smooth.

Nutritional Value (Amount per Serving):

- Calories 451
- Fat 34.2 g
- Carbohydrates 39.1 g
- Sugar 21.1 g
- Protein 4.8 g

Tropical Pineapple Orange Smoothie

Total Time: 5 minutes

Serves: 2

Ingredients:

- 1/2 cup pineapple chunks
- 4 tbsp coconut milk, unsweetened
- 3/4 cup fresh orange juice
- 6 tbsp vanilla yogurt
- 1/2 tbsp ground flax seed
- 1/2 banana

Directions:

1. Add all ingredients into the blender and blend until smooth.

Nutritional Value (Amount per Serving):

- Calories 200
- Fat 8.6 g
- Carbohydrates 27.2 g
- Sugar 19.7 g
- Protein 4.5 g
- Cholesterol 3 mg

Delicious Kale Banana Smoothie

Total Time: 5 minutes

Serves: 2

Ingredients:

- 2 cups kale, remove stems
- 1 banana
- 2 cups water
- 2 tbsp chia seeds
- 1/2 lime juice
- 2 cups pineapple chunks

Directions:

1. Add kale and water in blender and blend until smooth.
2. Now add remaining ingredients into the blender and blend again until smooth.
3. Serve immediately and enjoy.

Nutritional Value (Amount per Serving):

- Calories 168
- Fat 0.4 g
- Carbohydrates 42.1 g
- Sugar 23.5 g
- Protein 3.5 g
- Cholesterol 0 mg

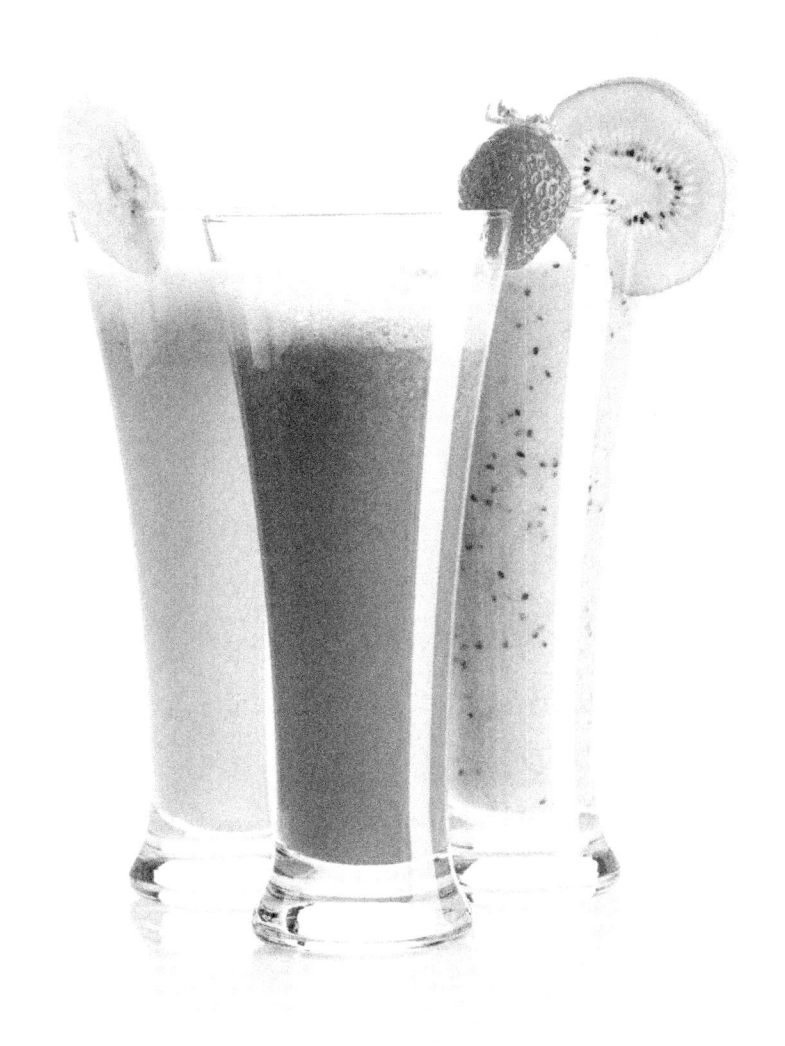

Easy Watermelon Strawberry Smoothie

Total Time: 5 minutes

Serves: 4

Ingredients:

- 4 cups watermelon chunks
- 2 cups strawberry
- 1 inch ginger
- 2 tbsp chia seeds
- 2 tbsp lime juice

Directions:

1. Add all ingredients into the blender and blend until smooth.

Nutritional Value (Amount per Serving):

- Calories 70
- Fat 0.5 g
- Carbohydrates 16.9 g
- Sugar 12.9 g
- Protein 1.4 g
- Cholesterol 0 mg

Energetic Lime Watermelon Smoothie

Total Time: 5 minutes

Serves: 2

Ingredients:

- 1 tbsp lime juice
- 2 cups watermelon chunks
- 3 fresh mint leaves
- 2 cups fresh strawberries

Directions:

1. Add all ingredients into the blender and blend until smooth.
2. Serve immediately and enjoy.

Nutritional Value (Amount per Serving):

- Calories 92
- Fat 0.6 g
- Carbohydrates 22.5 g
- Sugar 16.4 g
- Protein 1.9 g
- Cholesterol 0 mg

Zinger Papaya Ginger Smoothie

Total Time: 5 minutes

Serves: 4

Ingredients:

- 1 cup papaya chunks
- 1 inch ginger piece
- 3/4 cup milk
- 1 cup ice cube, crushed
- 1 cup pineapple chunks
- 1 tbsp lime juice
- 1 banana

Directions:

1. Add all ingredients into the blender and blend until smooth.
2. Serve immediately and enjoy.

Nutritional Value (Amount per Serving):

- Calories 85
- Fat 1.2 g
- Carbohydrates 18.3 g
- Sugar 12.5 g
- Protein 2.2 g
- Cholesterol 4 mg

Fresh Tropical Smoothie

Total Time: 5 minutes

Serves: 4

Ingredients:

- 1 cup papaya, cubed
- 4 cups almond milk
- 1 cup pineapple chunks
- 1/2 tbsp honey
- Ice

Directions:

1. Add all ingredients into the blender and blend until smooth.
2. Serve immediately and enjoy.

Nutritional Value (Amount per Serving):

- Calories 596
- Fat 57.4 g
- Carbohydrates 24.8 g
- Sugar 17.1 g
- Protein 5.9 g

Yummy Chocó Banana Smoothie

Total Time: 5 minutes

Serves: 4

Ingredients:

- 2 tsp cocoa powder
- 2 large bananas
- 1/2 cup ice cubes
- 2 tsp honey
- 1 1/2 cups milk

Directions:

1. Add all ingredients into the blender and blend until smooth and creamy.

Nutritional Value (Amount per Serving):

- Calories 119
- Fat 2.2 g
- Carbohydrates 23.4 g
- Sugar 15.3 g
- Protein 3.9 g
- Cholesterol 8 mg

Cool and Creamy Pumpkin Banana Smoothie

Total Time: 5 minutes

Serves: 2

Ingredients:

- 1 cup can pumpkin
- 1 banana
- Ground nutmeg
- 1 tsp pumpkin pie spice
- 6 ice cubes
- 1 cup almond milk
- 1 cup plain yogurt

Directions:

1. Add all ingredients except nutmeg into the blender and blend until smooth.
2. Garnish with ground nutmeg and serve.

Nutritional Value (Amount per Serving):

- Calories 460
- Fat 30.8 g
- Carbohydrates 39.2 g
- Sugar 24.0 g
- Protein 11.8 g
- Cholesterol 7 mg

Simple Mix Berry Smoothie

Total Time: 10 minutes

Serves: 2

Ingredients:

- 1 1/2 cup raspberries
- 3 kiwi, peeled and sliced
- 1 cup blueberries
- 2 cups orange juice
- 2 cups strawberries

Directions:

1. Add strawberries, blueberries and raspberries in blender and blend until smooth.
2. Then add orange juice and sliced kiwi and blend again until smooth.
3. Serve immediately and enjoy.

Nutritional Value (Amount per Serving):

- Calories 466
- Fat 1.6 g
- Carbohydrates 115.1 g
- Sugar 88.0 g
- Protein 4.9 g
- Cholesterol 0 mg

Healthy Immune Booster Smoothie

Total Time: 5 minutes

Serves: 2

Ingredients:

- 1/2 cup pineapple chunks
- 1 cup peaches
- 1 cup strawberries
- 1/2 cup plain yogurt
- 1 1/4 cups orange juice
- 6 ice cubes

Directions:

1. Add all ingredients into the blender and blend until smooth and creamy.

Nutritional Value (Amount per Serving):

- Calories 221
- Fat 1.3 g
- Carbohydrates 47.5 g
- Sugar 41.7 g
- Protein 5.5 g

Pink Grapefruit Raspberry Smoothie

Total Time: 5 minutes

Serves: 2

Ingredients:

- 2 grapefruit juice
- 2 cups fresh raspberries
- 2 fresh bananas

Directions:

1. Add all ingredients into the blender and blend until smooth.

Nutritional Value (Amount per Serving):

- Calories 210
- Fat 1.3 g
- Carbohydrates 52.0 g
- Sugar 28.8 g
- Protein 3.6 g
- Cholesterol 0 mg

Green Grape Avocado Smoothie

Total Time: 5 minutes

Serves: 2

Ingredients:

- 1/2 cup green grapes
- 1/2 avocado, remove seed and scoop out
- 1 banana
- 1 pear
- 2 tbsp chia seeds
- 2 cups water

Directions:

1. Add all ingredients into the blender and blend until smooth make sure chia seed nicely blend.

Nutritional Value (Amount per Serving):

- Calories 211
- Fat 10.2 g
- Carbohydrates 32.3 g
- Sugar 18.0 g
- Protein 2.0 g

Blueberry Chia Cherry Smoothie

Total Time: 5 minutes

Serves: 2

Ingredients:

- 1 cup fresh blueberries
- 4 tsp chia seeds
- 2 cups cherries, pitted
- 1 tbsp honey
- 2 cups coconut water

Directions:

1. Add all ingredients into the blender and blend until smooth.

Nutritional Value (Amount per Serving):

- Calories 145
- Fat 0.9 g
- Carbohydrates 36.2 g
- Sugar 29.8 g
- Protein 2.0 g
- Cholesterol 0 mg

Refreshing Apple Beet Smoothie

Total Time: 8 minutes

Serves: 4

Ingredients:

- 2 gala apple, diced
- 1 small beet, diced
- 1 cup filtered water
- 1 cup orange juice
- 12 ice cubes
- 1 1/2 cups fresh strawberries
- 3 tsp lemon juice
- 2 medium bananas

Directions:

1. Add all ingredients into the blender and blend until smooth.

Nutritional Value (Amount per Serving):

- Calories 145
- Fat 0.8 g
- Carbohydrates 34.7 g
- Sugar 24.1 g
- Protein 2.0 g
- Cholesterol 0 mg

Choco Cherry Smoothie

Total Time: 5 minutes

Serves: 2

Ingredients:

- 4 tbsp cocoa powder, unsweetened
- 2 cups cherries
- 2 cups almond milk, unsweetened
- 2 tbsp chia seeds
- 1/2 cup rolled oats
- 2 dates

Directions:

1. Add all ingredients into the blender and blend until smooth and creamy.

Nutritional Value (Amount per Serving):

- Calories 748
- Fat 60.7 g
- Carbohydrates 56.4 g
- Sugar 27.6 g
- Protein 11.8 g

Refreshing Melon Mint Smoothie

Total Time: 5 minutes

Serves: 2

Ingredients:

- 3 cups ripe honeydew melon
- 2 cup ice
- 20 mint leaves
- 5 tbsp lemon juice
- 1 tbsp honey
- 1 1/3 cup plain yogurt

Directions:

1. Add all ingredients into the blender and blend until smooth and creamy.
2. Serve and enjoy.

Nutritional Value (Amount per Serving):

- Calories 249
- Fat 2.7 g
- Carbohydrates 44.1 g
- Sugar 41.6 g
- Protein 11.0 g
- Cholesterol 10 mg

We thank you for reading, and hope this guide can be beneficial to you, in dealing with gout. We invite you to look up other related titles, including recipes on gout. Here are a few on the next page. We appreciate your reviews, & sharing your experiences with others. Everyone can benefit from everyone elses experiences.

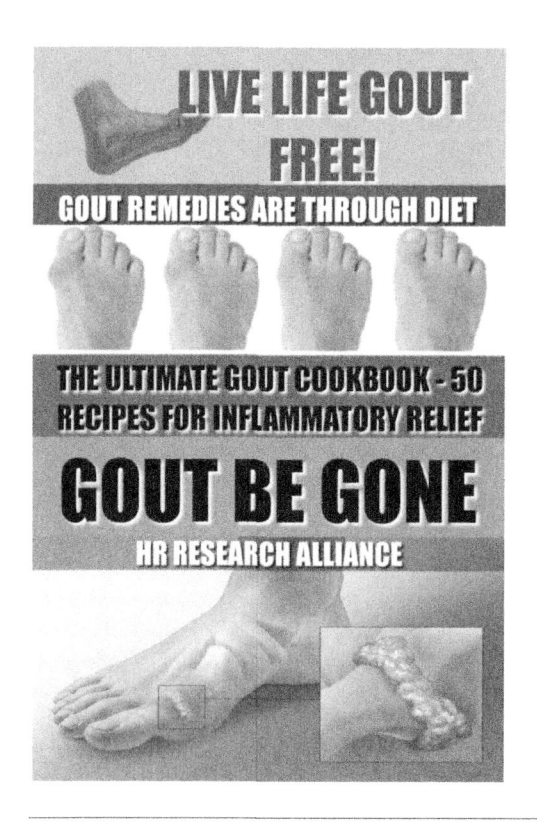

Gout
& ANTI INFLAMMATION MEAL PLAN GUIDE

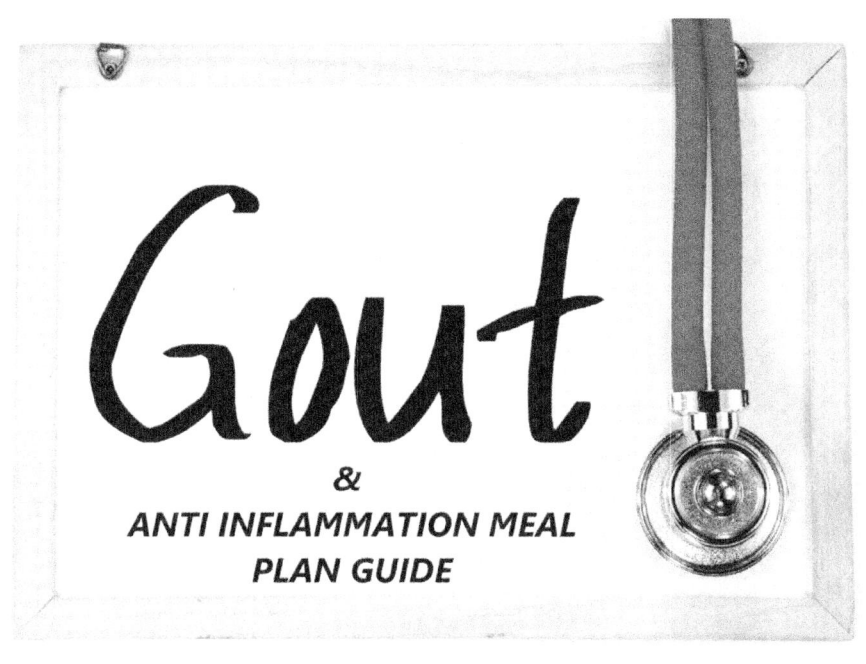

Nutritional Strategies For Reducing Inflammation Naturally

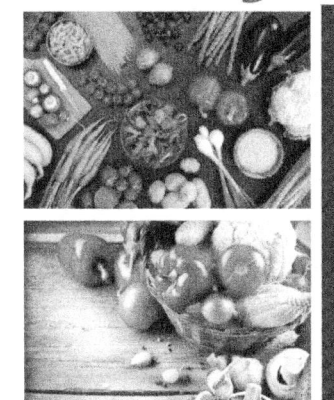

Gout Prevention - Gout Diet - Anti Inflammatory Foods To Eat & Avoid - & More...

HR Research Alliance

with 10 day meal plan & recipes

GOUT cookbook

cooking with SPICES for GOUT relief

HR Research Alliance

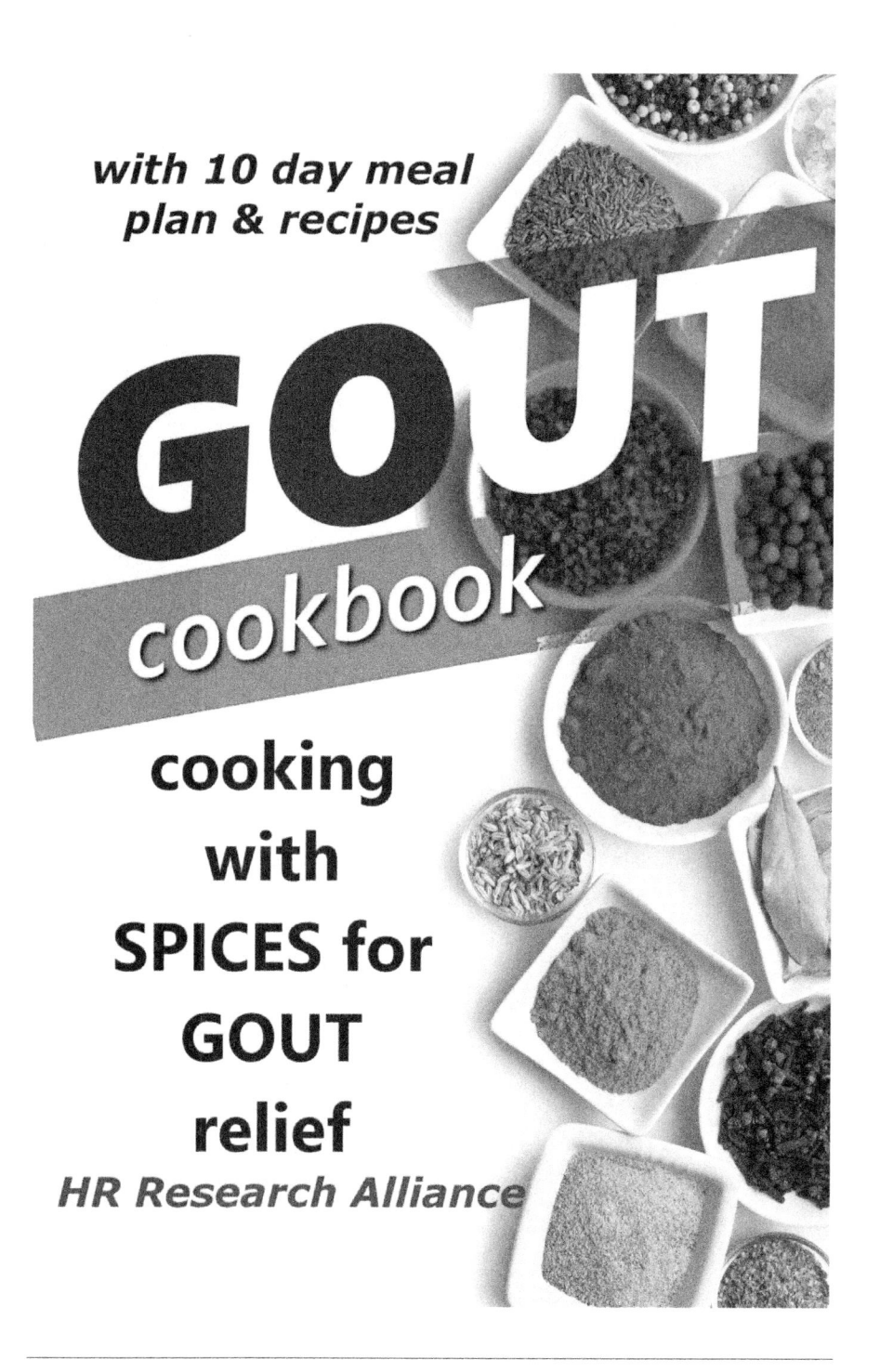

Disclaimer: All rights reserved. No part of this book may be reproduced or transmitted in any form or by any means, electronic or mechanical, including photocopying, recording or by any information storage and retrieval system, without written permission from the author, except for the inclusion of brief quotations in a review.The information provided in this book is designed to provide helpful information on the subjects discussed. This book is not meant to be used, nor should it be used, to diagnose or treat any medical condition. For diagnosis or treatment of any medical problem, consult your own physician. The publisher and author are not responsible for any specific health or allergy needs that may require medical supervision and are not liable for any damages or negative consequences from any treatment, action, application or preparation, to any person reading or following the information in this book.

References are provided for informational purposes only and do not constitute endorsement of any websites or other sources. Readers should be aware that the websites listed in this book may change.

This study aid is not intended to be any type of Medical advice. ALL individuals must consult their Doctors first and should always receive their meal plans from a qualified practitioner. . This book is not intended to heal, or cure anyone from any kind of illness, or disease.